# Reiki

*Unlocking the Secrets of Reiki Healing Aura Cleansing and Chakra Healing for Balancing Your Chakras, Including Guided Meditation Techniques to Reduce Stress*

© **Copyright 2019**

All rights Reserved. No part of this book may be reproduced in any form without permission in writing from the author. Reviewers may quote brief passages in reviews.

Disclaimer: No part of this publication may be reproduced or transmitted in any form or by any means, mechanical or electronic, including photocopying or recording, or by any information storage and retrieval system, or transmitted by email without permission in writing from the publisher.

While all attempts have been made to verify the information provided in this publication, neither the author nor the publisher assumes any responsibility for errors, omissions or contrary interpretations of the subject matter herein.

This book is for entertainment purposes only. The views expressed are those of the author alone, and should not be taken as expert instruction or commands. The reader is responsible for his or her own actions.

Adherence to all applicable laws and regulations, including international, federal, state and local laws governing professional licensing, business practices, advertising and all other aspects of doing business in the US, Canada, UK or any other jurisdiction is the sole responsibility of the purchaser or reader.

Neither the author nor the publisher assumes any responsibility or liability whatsoever on the behalf of the purchaser or reader of these materials. Any perceived slight of any individual or organization is purely unintentional

# Contents

INTRODUCTION ................................................................................................ 1

PART 1 - WHAT IS REIKI? ................................................................................ 3

CHAPTER 1: PRINCIPLES OF REIKI ................................................................. 4
    *Meaning of Reiki* ........................................................................................ 4
    *Universal Life Force Channel* ..................................................................... 5
    *The Process of Giving and Receiving* ........................................................ 5
    *Chakras and the Endocrine System* .......................................................... 6
    *Subtle Chakras of the Hands and Feet* ..................................................... 9
    *Auras* ........................................................................................................ 10
    *Attunements* ........................................................................................... 13
    *Degrees: First, Second, and Third* ........................................................... 14
    *Reiki Principles* ........................................................................................ 15
    *Reiki Is for Everyone* ............................................................................... 16
    *Benefits* .................................................................................................... 16

CHAPTER 2: ORIGINS OF REIKI .................................................................... 19
    *Buddhism and Reiki* ................................................................................ 19
    *Japanese Origins* ..................................................................................... 20
    *Western Origins* ...................................................................................... 21
    *Modern Practice* ..................................................................................... 22
    *Kundalini and Ki, Chi, Prana, Light* .......................................................... 23
    *Mind, Body, Spirit, Wholeness* ................................................................ 26

PART 2: THE FIRST DEGREE ......................................................................... 28

CHAPTER 3: PURPOSE OF THE FIRST DEGREE ........................................... 29
    *Attunements* ........................................................................................... 29

  *Self-Healing* ............................................................................ *30*

## CHAPTER 4: HAND POSITIONS ............................................. 32
  *Ending a Self-Treatment* ...................................................... *37*
  *Healing Common Ailments* ................................................... *38*

## CHAPTER 5: PRACTICE HEALING OTHERS ........................... 40
  *Preparing to Treat Others* ..................................................... *41*
  *Invocation* ............................................................................ *43*
  *The Treatment Experience* .................................................... *44*
  *Hand Positions for Treating Others* ....................................... *47*
  *Express Reiki Treatment* ....................................................... *52*

## CHAPTER 6: OTHER APPLICATIONS WITH REIKI IN THE FIRST DEGREE ............. 55
  *Solfeggio Frequencies* ........................................................... *55*
  *Reiki and Animals* ................................................................ *57*
  *Reiki in the Garden* .............................................................. *58*

## CHAPTER 7: CONCLUSION OF THE FIRST DEGREE ............... 59

## PART 3: THE SECOND DEGREE .............................................. 61

## CHAPTER 8: PURPOSE OF THE SECOND DEGREE ................. 62

## CHAPTER 9: PILLARS OF REIKI .............................................. 65
  *First Pillar: Gassho* ............................................................... *65*
  *Second Pillar: Reiji-Ho* .......................................................... *67*
  *Third Pillar: Chiryo* .............................................................. *68*
  *Practicing Pillars of Reiki* ..................................................... *70*

## CHAPTER 10: THE SACRED REIKI SYMBOLS ......................... 71
  *Why Learn and Use the Symbols?* ......................................... *72*
  *Three Main Uses of Reiki Symbols* ........................................ *73*
  *Preparing to Draw the Symbols* ............................................ *73*
  *The First Symbol: Cho Ku Rei* ............................................... *74*
  *The Second Symbol: Sei Heiki* .............................................. *76*
  *The Third Symbol: Hon Sha Ze Sho Nen* ............................... *78*

## CHAPTER 11: DISTANCE HEALING ........................................ 83
  *Preparations for Reiki Distance Healing* ............................... *84*
  *Methods for Sending Distance Healing* ................................. *86*
  *Techniques for Visualization* ................................................. *89*
  *Traditional Distance Healing Technique* ............................... *90*
  *Example Uses for Distance Healing* ...................................... *91*

**CHAPTER 12: CONCLUSION OF THE SECOND DEGREE ............... 95**

**PART 4: THE THIRD DEGREE ............... 97**

**CHAPTER 13: PURPOSE OF THE THIRD DEGREE ............... 98**

**CHAPTER 14: UNDERSTANDING THE POWER OF SYMBOLS ............... 100**

*Symbols in Reiki ............... 102*

**CHAPTER 15: REIKI MASTER SYMBOL ............... 104**

*Dai Ko Myo ............... 104*
*Nontraditional Master Symbols ............... 107*

**CHAPTER 16: ATTUNING STUDENTS TO USE REIKI ............... 108**

*Simple Rules for Attuning Others ............... 108*
*Steps for the Attunement: First Degree ............... 109*
*Steps for Attunement: Second Degree ............... 112*
*Steps for Attunement: Third Degree ............... 113*
*Steps for Combination Attunement: First, Second, and Third Degrees ...... 113*
*Crown to Crown Attunement ............... 114*
*Absent or Distant Attunements ............... 114*
*Psychic Surgery ............... 116*

**CHAPTER 17: CONCLUSION OF THE THIRD DEGREE ............... 120**

**CONCLUSION ............... 122**

# Introduction

Today, our society sees health concerns through the lens of surgery, drugs, and prescriptions given by medical caregivers. Technology encourages our advancement to improve the medical industry, so it can give people what they need.

Yet, in our knowledge and discovery, the ancient healing energies of Universal Life Force have always existed; it is free, and it is for everyone. It can cure and balance any ailment of the body, mind, and spirit.

Why are we not using these healing energies every day? The time is here to acknowledge your inner wisdom and healing power. Anyone living can perform this healing technique to cure health concerns, sickness, colds, injuries, chronic and acute disorders, mental health, emotional imbalances, and so much more.

The ancient healing technique known as Reiki has been a part of our knowledge for over two thousand years, possibly even earlier. It can open your earthly life to the limitless bounty of healing energy that exists in all things.

Once you are attuned to the power of channeling Reiki energy, you can utilize this energy to heal yourself, your family and friends, and anything you touch. The possibilities are limitless!

This book will give you instruction on how to enrich your life with the power of Universal Life Force. Connecting your senses with the energy of your soul to bring healing into the world, you can master the techniques of Reiki and invite balance, well-being, and harmony into your everyday life.

You will learn a variety of techniques, meditations, hand-positions for channeling Reiki, as well as how it works, why it works, and the way it benefits all things in life.

Today's society is changing and so is our understanding of what we are capable. Anyone can bring this light and energy into their hands for healing.

Reiki is in you. Bring it forward and heal yourself, your life, and anyone who wants to understand its healing power.

# Part 1 - What Is Reiki?

# Chapter 1: Principles of Reiki

Your existence on earth isn't just matter and physical reality. There are energies within us and all around us that are always shifting and impacting our life experience. This knowledge isn't secret; it has been studied, examined, contemplated, and practiced by many human beings throughout history. Much of what is known about Reiki and its healing powers comes from ancient texts and a handful of masters, but before we dig into the origins, let's begin with some of the basics of what Reiki is and how it works.

## Meaning of Reiki

Reiki is a combination of two Japanese characters that embody the essence of what *Reiki* means. The word *Rei* means "Universal" and the word *ki* means "life force." The two together create the concept of *Universal Life Force*. This describes the energy that exists in all things in the universe and simply states what kind of energy is being channeled. Even though the original writings about Reiki were written in Sanskrit within Buddhist texts, the name given to the practice was given by a Japanese monk who was called to bring the knowledge of this ancient healing power to the modern world.

## Universal Life Force Channel

The concept of Reiki is available to everyone because it exists in and around everyone. That is what it means to be universal. You are not given a gift of healing power, rather you are opened and attuned to the Universal Life Force energies and act as a channel of this energy to empower healing in others.

You do not heal the person receiving Reiki; they heal themselves as you channel this energy through your hands and direct it into their bodies and auras. The energy travels to where the body needs it most and provides healing.

## The Process of Giving and Receiving

Once you are attuned to the Reiki energy through degrees of learning and practice, your hands become a conduit for the healing energy so that it may pass through you for specific areas of healing or into the body and energy system of another.

There are several specific hand positions, symbols, and techniques that allow you to provide Reiki energy to anything. Your hands are the gateway for sending energy out of you and into another. In this process, you do not interact with the ailments of another or acquire any of their illness, rather you send energy through yourself and into the places that need attention and focus into the receiver.

The process is healing for both the giver and the receiver, as you will both become connected to the Universal Life Force energy. As you slowly shift and move your hand positions across your own or another person's body, you empower the already existing energy for replenishment, revitalization, and balance.

A full body Reiki session can last an hour to an hour and a half because your movements are very slow. Each hand position and energy channeling should last between three and five minutes.

Part of the healing session involves combing and cleansing the aura before and after. All Reiki healing uses the hands for channeling energy into the body.

## Chakras and the Endocrine System

Your Reiki healing experience is directly linked to your **chakras**, or main energy centers, and your endocrine system, the system in your body that contains all of your glands which regulate hormone function and other chemical performances to keep the body in balance.

There are seven main chakras that go from the root located at the base of your spine, and out through the top of your head. Each chakra connects to specific organ and body functions, emotions, colors, and healing processes. Since you are working with healing the energy of your whole system, it is important to know what this energy is and how it connects to your well-being.

> 1. **The Root Chakra:** The root chakra is red and is located at the base of the spine. It represents physical vitality, creation, birth, security, and life. It is here that your Kundalini energy is coiled before it awakens on a journey to spiritual enlightenment. The root is connected to the spine, kidneys, bladder, and renal glands.
> A balanced root chakra feels secure, abundant, centered, calm, grounded, and connected to nature and the earth.
> Emotional imbalance here feels like insecurity, anger, depression, nervousness, greed, and unnecessary fear. Physical imbalance here shows as frequent illness, obesity, eating disorders, knee troubles, and hip discomfort.
> 2. **The Sacral Chakra:** The sacral chakra is orange and located below the navel, above the root chakra. It represents sexual energy, first impressions of others, and perceptions. It is associated with the legs, reproductive organs, and the reproductive glands.

With a balanced sacral chakra, you will feel joyful, creative, passionate, and capable of connecting physically with another person.

Emotional imbalance in the sacral chakra may feel like unworthiness, feeling of isolation, numbness, stiff or cold emotions, and overly sensitive. Physical imbalance can manifest as sexual addiction, inhibited sexual desire, or hormone imbalance, and brings a potential for miscarriages and difficulty conceiving.

3. **The Solar Plexus Chakra:** The solar plexus is yellow and is positioned just above the navel. This is the center of your body and is the place where food is converted to energy and distributed throughout the body. It is connected to vitality and power, supplied energy, emotions, and the digestive system including the stomach, liver, and pancreas.

Balance in this chakra gives the feeling of energy and drive, confidence, active and cheerful disposition, and a strong sense of purpose.

Sometimes, imbalance here looks like alternate sides of the same coin: arrogant demeanor, demanding attitude, overbearing sensibilities, and addictions versus deficiency of energy, feelings of helplessness, weakness, timidity, or submissiveness.

4. **The Heart Chakra:** The heart chakra is affiliated with the color green and sometimes rosy pink. It is the place of emotion, love, connection, compassion, spiritual growth, and openness to all living things.

A balanced heart chakra exudes Universal love, compassion, interconnectedness, acceptance, and harmony from within one's being.

As with the solar plexus chakra, imbalance here can manifest as excessiveness or deficiency. Deficiency in the heart feels low self-esteem, sadness, isolation, depression, and shortness of breath. Excess energy in the heart chakra looks like codependency, clingy behavior, and superfluous care taking of others.

**5. The Throat Chakra:** The throat chakra is a light blue in color and is the seat of self-expression, communication, emotional expression, and creativity. Energy goes to the thyroid, upper lungs, arms, and digestive tract, through the esophagus.

A balance of energy here appears as good communication, honest self-expression, emotional articulation and clarity, and creativity.

Emotional imbalances or blockages can manifest as suppressed emotions, difficulty expressing feelings, and an inability to release old trauma and wounds from past experiences. Physical imbalance can show up as sore throat, difficulty hearing and inner ear problems, stiff neck and shoulders, and stagnant creative flow.

**6. The Third Eye (Brow Chakra):** The third eye is located at the brow line and is indigo. This is the center of psychic perception, vision, telepathy, and Extrasensory Perception. This chakra supplies energy to the spine, lower brain, pituitary gland, left eye, ears, and central nervous system.

Balance here enhances perception, improved memory and cognitive ability, displays comfort with the force of life and death, creates a strong connection to your intuition, and clairvoyant and telepathic abilities.

An imbalance in the third eye can manifest as headaches, mental health issues and illness, hallucinations and nightmares, paranoia, anxiety, and delusions. It can also be connected to the health of your physical eyes, so healing of the eyes is important.

**7. The Crown Chakra:** The crown chakra is on the top of your head and is either white or violet. It is the entrance point of the Universal Life Force that you channel through your being. This energy supplies the pineal gland, right eye, and upper brain.

Balance here is expanded consciousness, transcendence, understanding and acceptance of the immortality of the soul, increased spiritual gifts and capabilities, and the creation of miracles, such as channeling Reiki energy for healing.

Imbalances and blockages here can manifest as migraines, headaches, and head tension, boredom, apathy or disconnectedness, and an inability to comprehend or retain new knowledge.

## Subtle Chakras of the Hands and Feet

Although not considered any of the main chakras, the energy centers on the palms of your hands and soles of your feet are of significant importance in Reiki healing and general whole-body balance and wellness.

As you attune to channeling Reiki, your hands will become a significant part of the experience. It is through the hands that you pass the power of Reiki into another. You will also feel the warmth of energy around all things with your hands. Your hands will be in balance with this energy as all of your other energy centers harmonize and you receive Reiki attunement.

Your feet are also significant energy centers; they ground you to the earth and help direct your whole energy flow. You will notice the energy at the soles of the feet more as you open and attune. You will understand how powerful grounding to the earth is once you feel that energetic power.

All of the chakras work together to bring balance and harmony to your life. When we have imbalances, we suffer from emotional and physical ailment, sometimes chronic. These imbalances can even lead to disease. Eastern culture has been practicing awareness and healing of these subtle energies for centuries. It is only in the recent past that Western culture has begun to include more of this knowledge in its healing and health practices. Even with our advanced technology and ability to share information worldwide, so many societies and cultures haven't fully embraced the universal true of our energy systems and health.

Reiki works with this energy, clearing and balancing the chakras of the body to prevent illness and promote wellness.

## Auras

The auras are a part of the self that are energy fields surrounding your physical form. Each field of energy extends from your body in colorful layers, all connected to different aspects of the internal energy and life force. They often look a certain color when seen by aura light detecting photography. Depending on the colors, you can identify characteristics of your mind, body, and spirit condition.

As there are seven main chakras, there are also seven auric fields. You can identify the qualities of the auric fields with the seven chakras. From the closest to your skin to the outermost aura, they are as follows:

1. **Etheric (1st):** The first aura is only about 1 to 5 centimeters from your skin. It is connected to the root chakra energy but has a bluish-grey color. Of all the auras, it is usually the easiest to detect with the naked eye. It connects to your physical form: muscles, bones, tissues, fascia, etc. It has a slower pulse or vibration than the other auras.
A weak etheric aura is usually caused by inactivity, lack of exercise, or connection to your body through some kind of motion. Immunity can be compromised when this aura is weak. It can be healed through fitness, exercise, dance, walking, being in nature, hiking, and various other activities.

2. **Emotional (2nd):** The next aura extends out from the skin about 2 to 5 centimeters. It is connected to your sacral chakra and can appear as any and all colors of the rainbow. The shape of this aura is exactly like the shape of the first aura. Some say, it looks like soft, colorful clouds, constantly in motion like our emotions often are. If you are experiencing

emotional upheaval, blockages, or stress, this aura can appear muddled or frozen.

All of your emotions are represented here (anger, love, doubt, worry, hope, fear, joy, etc.) and the state of all your chakras can be determined from this auric field. It is an essential part of manifestation and action in your life.

3. **Mental (3rd):** At a higher vibration, the mental aura is connected to your solar plexus chakra, as well as your thoughts, cognition, ego, and personal power. It extends from the physical body about 6 to 10 centimeters. Like the chakra associated with it, this auric field is bright yellow and radiates strongest around the head, neck, and shoulders. It will appear strongest in those who are often engaged in mental tasks or overactive thought. Some have reported seeing sparks of color flowing from this aura during creative moments.

The character of your thoughts will color this aura and display the emotional quality of your thoughts. For example, if your thoughts tend to be darker, then you may have a dimmer coloring to this yellow aura. It can be activated through teaching or learning, research, reading, and specific kinds of meditation and energy stimulation, such as Reiki.

4. **Astral (4th):** Rosy pink in hue, and represented by the heart chakra, the astral aura is directly connected to the capacity for conditional and unconditional love. It extends from the physical body 15 to 30 centimeters and is where we form our "cords of connection" with others, whether they are positive or negative. This aura is strengthened by intimacy and loving, healing relationships. It is weakened by conflicts, break-ups, and trauma related to partnership. Like the emotional (2nd) aura, the astral aura appears like beautifully pink-colored clouds. Discoloration reflects the current state of the heart center.

The astral aura is the opening to the astral and angelic world. It also acts as the bridge between the lower (denser) auras and the upper (lighter) auras. This is the realm of emotional experience, dreams, fantasies, astral projection, visions, near-death experience, and imagination.

5. **Etheric Double (5th):** The first aura is also called the etheric body and relates to the physical properties of the self. The 5th aura is a mirror, or double of the first aura, and is connected to the heart chakra. It is the entire blueprint of your body and contains everything you create including your personality, identity, and general energy.

It is between 30 and 60 centimeters from the skin and is blue or cobalt in color, though it can also be in various colors. It is activated by sound and can be awakened through certain sound therapies. It also can be healed or recharged when you speak your truth and is strengthened when you know your true self.

6. **Celestial (6th):** The celestial aura is connected to the brow chakra, or third eye, which represents higher intellect, wisdom, collective consciousness, and psychic/spiritual openness. It has a very powerful vibration in comparison to the other auras and connects you to the Divine and all beings. Feelings of oneness, awareness, creative visualization, and life purpose are prominent in this aura.

This aura is a pearly white color and extends 80 to 90 centimeters from the physical body. It is difficult to see with the naked eye, but they say this aura has pastel colors mixed with silver-gold light beams, giving off a pearly-white or mother of pearl quality. It is stimulated and strengthened through meditation and spiritual transformation.

7. **Causal (7th):** Furthest from the physical body, extended out 2 to 3 feet, the causal aura is the seat of divine consciousness and the plan of your soul. Information about your past lives and soul contracts for your current incarnation are held here, like the soul's history and design. It is golden and has the highest vibration frequency of all the auras, pulsating at a very rapid rate.

The causal body is egg-shaped, like it is containing the other six auras in a shell of golden protection. It is stimulated by certain kinds of meditation, but is also greatly affected, opened, and attuned to energy healing, such as Reiki. When it is strong, it will help you surrender to your life path and can also facilitate connection to the divine and other psychic and clairvoyant experiences.

## Attunements

When you give or receive Reiki, you are transmitting channeled energy that exists in all things. It is the initiation of healing energy that brings your body, mind, and spirit into balance. This is one of the most important parts of learning and understanding Reiki.

These transmissions are known in Reiki as attunements. An attunement touches the energy of the etheric body and releases the mental, emotional, and physical toxins within a person. It's like tuning into a certain radio frequency that beams healing energy waves through your hands into another person's being.

The person giving the Reiki treatment channels the energy through their crown chakra, down the arms and into the hands. Once the charge of energy can be felt in the hands, the Reiki practitioner can now offer healing to himself or herself and others.

Each degree of attunement follows specific hand positions, symbols, and mantras known to the Reiki practitioner. The knowledge of these attunement symbols and techniques is most often passed from the Reiki teacher to the student in the first attunement. Once you have become 'attuned' and learned the symbols and hand positions, you can perform Reiki healing treatment on yourself and others.

People describe different sensations when they are being attuned to Reiki, such as waves of energy, warmth, or coldness, some see colorful light and may feel tingling sensations throughout the body. Your first attunement can sometimes have certain side-affects, like headache, exhaustion, and other symptoms. This is usually a good sign that your body is clearing toxins and is healing itself.

In order to be awakened to this energy, it is suggested that you see a Reiki practitioner who can give your first attunement, which is what opens you up the First Degree of Reiki healing.

## Degrees: First, Second, and Third

The Reiki training techniques are divided into three degrees. The degrees are essentially levels of learning and opening to the Reiki energy. Each degree encapsulates specific meditations that are conducted by a teacher, or master, who teaches you the background of Reiki and all its benefits.

- **The First Degree:** This is your first, real experience with this powerful energy. It is in this degree that you are officially attuned. You will learn the history and origins of Reiki, hand positions for healing, benefits of Reiki, and how to work on giving yourself healing treatments.
This is the level of healing the self before healing others. It opens up your upper four chakras (crown, brow, throat, and heart) to prepare you to receive Reiki. You will also feel a release and balancing between all of your chakras and whole system. Once you are an opened channel, it will never close again. You will always have the ability to connect to Universal Life Force energy. The more you use it, the stronger it becomes. Daily use for three weeks to three months is encouraged in the First Degree before moving into the Second Degree.
- **The Second Degree:** In here, you have already been attuned and have practiced healing yourself for at least a month. You may have even performed some Reiki treatments for friends, family, or pets.
This level teaches more focused methods for handling deeply emotional issues and mental traumas. Here, you will deepen your connection to your intuition, subconscious,

superconscious, and higher self. You will strengthen your healing powers and learn more advanced ways of healing and transforming negative behavior patterns, addictions, depressions, and many more severe ailments.

This degree also opens you to the ability to perform long-distance Reiki healing. In this technique, you can beam Reiki energy across great distances directly to a receiver.

This attunement is significantly more powerful than the first and holds greater responsibility for a practitioner.

• **The Third Degree:** This final degree is called the Master degree. If you are interested in making Reiki a way of life and practicing it as a vocation to heal and teach people, then the third level will be something to pursue. It can take someone one to three years by traditional Reiki standards to achieve mastery.

Here, you will experience a higher level of spiritual maturity, substantial personal growth on all levels, and mastery of life overall. This degree requires the greatest responsibility of all three levels and will put you in the position to train new masters as you continue providing healing attunements.

## Reiki Principles

Reiki is a healing practice, not a religion, but it contains within it some basic principles to live by and to attune to as you engage in the Universal Life Force energy. The principles are basic, and it is recommended as you begin your healing journey that you memorize or carry with you a few principles. They are:

Just for today, I will not worry.

Just for today, I will not be angry.

Just for today, I will do my work honestly.

Just for today, I will give thanks for my many blessings.

Just for today, I will be kind to every living thing.

These principles, simply stated, describe the essentials of living a whole and balanced life. As you become attuned to your energy and healing abilities, you will need to concentrate on the benefits of these principles. They are small ideas that speak volumes about those who choose to practice them.

## Reiki Is for Everyone

Many people view Reiki as a practice reserved for only certain people: gifted healers, practitioners of Eastern philosophies, and gurus. The essence of Reiki is that it is built around the concept of universal energy that exists in all living things. We all have the ability to channel Reiki—men, women, and even children!

Whole families will sometimes learn together so that they can help each other in healing processes and through difficult times. There are great benefits to sharing these skills with children because they can learn a deeper understanding of themselves and also walk through the world with greater calm and centeredness.

The possibilities are limitless with Reiki, and everyone can learn these techniques. You can simply learn them to heal yourself and leave it at that. You can move through the degrees toward mastery, if you feel that it is your calling.

Reiki, as a part of everyday life, has boundless potential to improve not just you and your family or friends, but everyone. If we all come together to learn and teach this universal skill, think of how different the world would be.

Reiki comes to those who are ready for it, and maybe you can be the one to open the door to others who want to cross the threshold to healing and harmony.

## Benefits

Since its entrance into modern culture, Reiki has shown significant promise in the healing of many ailments. Not only does it give offerings to the soul and an essence of energetic health and wellbeing, it also acts as an antidote to many diseases, illnesses, discomforts, and injustices of the intellect and heart.

Thoughts and feelings, when felt through negative filters and past traumas, accrue imbalances in all of the chakras. The discomfort of these negative beliefs, ideas, and sensations of the self can develop into problems of the heart, mind, and body.

Reiki clears and dissolves so much that may lead to disease. Benefits of allowing Reiki healing to come into you are numerous and some of the most commonly reported effects are as follows:

- Brings about a sense of security, calm, and beauty in the soul
- Alleviates patterns of doubt and distress
- Awakens the soul to the true light self
- Brings forth all insecurities for purging and healing
- Stimulates channels of the chakras and endocrine system for alignment and health
- Destroys elements of sickness and helps aid the body in re-discovering internal healing power
- Opens the eye of the mind to witness and perceive the world, the self, and others with clear sight
- Connects you to the Earth and opens the angelic realm
- Reduces anger, hate, distrust, and discouragement
- Changes your inner world to exist in harmony and love with your outer world
- Dispels diseases such as cancer, tumors, lymphoma, AIDS, chronic, and acute illnesses
- Expunges thoughts, attitudes, and histories of pain and fear
- Penetrates the essence of any issue to allow for all healing possibilities
- And so much more…

There isn't anything holding you back from knowing the truth of your energy and the rise of Reiki inside of your life. Let's get in touch with all of the lessons you can go through to become attuned to Reiki in your life.

# Chapter 2: Origins of Reiki

Beyond time, there is nothing but life force. The entrance of intuition into the energies that heal was not written about or described until rather recently in our human history, although 'healing powers' were not unheard of in the annals of human experience.

Facts and dates about the healing energy we now call Reiki reach back to roughly two thousand years before the age of Buddha, but who knows how long we have described and understood this life force as humans. The work of certain philosophers and agents of truth brought the rules and doctrines of this method of healing into focus in the world not so long ago. This chapter brings to light a tale of tradition, knowledge, and the magic of healing.

## Buddhism and Reiki

Buddha is widely recognized throughout our entire global system of religion. He is considered the Godfather of Holiness and honors the tradition of attuning to the internal light and being for the purpose of existing with wholeness. The practices created as a result of

Buddha's determination to follow his intuition and gain clarity brought our world into a sense of understanding regarding the source of enlightenment on our planet.

Within the teachings of Buddhism, you can connect any and all dots to an idea of energy inside the soul. When in honor of light and love, this the power to create miracles and open the Earth to a connective, collective consciousness.

In the sacred Vedic texts of ancient Hindu belief, there were scriptures pertaining to our life force energy. These texts likely influenced Buddha, who succumbed to a journey of enlightenment through the words, intentions, ideas, and methods outlined in these texts, describing the Universal Life Force and how it can bless the Earth's souls. When he learned of this energy he acted upon it to offer healing lessons to others but wasn't able to design the structure of these techniques.

Their condition remained blanketed in other sacred texts and teachings without any true form for giving knowledge of this gift to others. It remained in an archive of Hindu and Buddhist doctrine that taught the knowledge of this energetic power to followers of this religion and no one else.

## Japanese Origins

Beyond Buddha, and hundreds of years later in the beginning of the 20$^{th}$ century, a man called Mikao Usui was living as a Buddhist monk. As a monk, meditations that last for days and even weeks were not uncommon. For Usui, a 21-day meditation and fast brought him directly into the path of an awakening that would give birth to Reiki.

The story goes that, while in his meditation high on a mountain, he was pondering the concepts he had studied in the Buddhist texts, in which the concept of energy systems in the body and healing power are described. In one telling of the story, he committed to this quest for knowing the source of our healing power before becoming a monk. To help some missionary students answer the question of the possibility of healing others as Christ had, Usui was determined to find answers.

While he dedicated himself to uncovering the secret truths of a Universal Life Force, he spent the last days of his meditation looking for the answer within himself. All of a sudden, he felt as though he was struck by lightning in his third eye, opening his awareness and awakening his soul. This profound moment brought him the answer he sought. He scurried down the mountain, stubbing his toe along the way, but as it bled, he cupped his hands around the wound and caused the bleeding to stop and the pain to dissolve.

The details of this tale remain uncertain. According to Reiki tradition, the story of Usui is passed down from Master teacher to pupil, so the story now has many versions.

He decided to dedicate his life to teaching and healing using his awakened understanding of this energy and its power. Inspired by the sacred Buddhist texts, Usui created to a version of this energy practice we know today as Reiki.

He trained many students, but no one was a master except for his successor, Dr. Chijiro Hayashi, who had worked side-by-side with Usui and mastered the art of Reiki under the original master.

## Western Origins

Before WWII, a Japanese woman living in Hawaii named Hawayo Takata was living a life of misery. She had experienced significant losses in her family and suffered from nervous exhaustion which led to severe sickness, disease, and tumors that required an operation. It is said that when Takata was about to go into surgery, she heard a voice in her head that explained that her surgery was not necessary. She heeded the voice's warning to leave the surgery and found herself back in Japan at the Reiki clinic established by Usui. She stayed there for months and healed completely from all of her disease, tumor, and overall ill health. She decided to stay and become a Reiki practitioner and received training at the clinic before returning home to Hawaii to establish her own Reiki practice.

Eventually, she became the next master after Hayashi and, up to that point, there were few masters but many students. Around this time, her granddaughter and a woman doctor studied under her and both became masters, at which point, freedom was given to teach mastery to anyone willing and open to making Reiki a part of his or her life.

Since then, Reiki has expanded in Western culture, but saw a decline in Japan after WWII and has only recently begun to revive there. Reiki was kept alive in the West and has been passed through many Masters.

The concept of Reiki is handed down in specific ways from Master to the pupil, but over the years, each practitioner loosens the original concepts a little more. The essence of Reiki practice remains the same, but because so many of the original teachings were kept a secret and only revealed in teachings with a Master, so much of the original Japanese Reiki may have been lost or altered through time.

What hasn't changed is Reiki itself. Nothing changes our ability to understand the healing of ourselves and others through this energy. We may need guidance along the road, but once Reiki is attuned in you, it never goes away.

## Modern Practice

Today's Reiki culture is now worldwide with more and more people becoming attuned every year. Original practices meant that it took several years to go through the degrees in order to prove you are ready to take on the responsibility of being a Reiki Master. More recently, you can take a weekend workshop and receive the initial and second-degree attunements to engage your system before you go off in the world to practice.

There are thousands of websites, blog posts, videos, and teachers all over the world that are revealing the happiness and healing that comes from opening to this energy. It is more accessible than ever and even though there are sources that say you must follow a certain protocol to learn Reiki, there will always be your own knowing of what works best for you.

This book is a great resource for modern Reiki practitioners because it embraces the original and the new to show you how valuable your life can become when you open yourself to your healing potential.

## Kundalini and Ki, Chi, Prana, Light

The philosophy behind Reiki has much older origins than the turn of the 20$^{th}$ century and comes from many Eastern cultures, not just Japan. As you study Reiki and the essences of these techniques, you will find common links across Eastern cultures that shed light on the same search for truth and enlightenment.

Universal Light Force energy, the throbbing, pulsing hum that lives within all beings, is everywhere and available to everyone. Each philosophy or religion explains it in different terms and through a different language, yet the essential things are the same. We can all open to the healing energy of the universe and can channel it through our being for healing.

Understanding some of the other names for this energy, or how it has influenced other cultures, is important to opening yourself to the collective harmony of life in all things. We may come from different backgrounds and speak different languages, but we all share this energy. Call it as you desire; Reiki is universal and brings us together to bring balance to humanity with love and healing.

- **Kundalini Rising**
  
  The origins of Kundalini date back as early as Reiki. The Sanskrit texts that mention the universal healing energy within also mentioned the concept of Kundalini. Are they the same? Kundalini concepts appeared in the Vedas of Hindu religious texts and described the internal subtle energy bodies (chakras), and how they are awakened to begin the journey toward enlightenment.

Many of the modern Kundalini practices are tied to a specific branch of yoga of the same name that inspires the awakening of this dormant energy within the body. According to sources who have experienced Kundalini awakening, it is not always ignited through yoga practices. For some, it awakens spontaneously due to traumatic life events, challenging emotional upheavals, chronic illnesses, or diseases.

The basic idea behind Kundalini is that from the time you are conceived in this world, you have a coil of life that has sparked at the base of your spine. This word *Kundalini* translates to mean "coiled up," but once awakened, it rises through the body, purging and cleansing all of the chakras all the way up through the crown and usually back down to the root to complete the journey of enlightenment.

The purging and cleansing of the chakras can elicit many physical and emotional reactions that require devotion to awaken so that you may balance your energy and experience inner peace and harmony.

It is important to note that in Kundalini texts, it is made clear that every person alive has Kundalini, but not every person will awaken their energy in their lifetime.

Much like Reiki, this Universal Life Force can be accessed with the right circumstances and conditions to awaken the soul and spirit. The difference, however, is that Kundalini is about the awakening of the true self to give love and light to the world. Reiki opens your channels and chakras so that you may heal yourself and others. There isn't any focus on Kundalini being used as a tool to help people connect to the channel of healing energy, only that it awakens you to your own healing to reach enlightenment.

In Reiki, you experience an awakening, and although it may not manifest in the same way that is described in Kundalini, your whole system must go through change, purging, cleansing, and healing to live in harmony with this energy. It is possible that when you become attuned to Reiki for the first time, you light the fire of Kundalini awakening, beginning your whole healing journey through cycles of attunement.

For the Reiki practitioner, it may be helpful to do more research on Kundalini and the effects of awakening that life force.

- **Ki, Qi, Prana, Light**

Across cultures and Eastern philosophies, there are different words to describe the same energetic life force that we all possess and can attune to: Qi (chi), Prana, Light (Holy Spirit). The difference between them is simply borders, cultural boundaries, and religious differences.

*Ki* is the Japanese word you learned earlier in Chapter 1 to describe the part of Reiki that means "life force." A very similar sounding word, Qi (Chi), comes from the Chinese philosophies and healing traditions. Such traditions describe the same life force or 'vital energy' that is within everyone and requires balance and healing through the use of herbal remedy, healing diet, and physical and mental meditation practices, such as the concept of Tai Chi and Chi Gong. The origins of Qi in Chinese medicine have ancient and early roots, like the understanding of Ki through sacred Buddhist texts.

The Hindu traditions and culture refer to this Universal Life Force as 'Prana.' Its literal translation is 'life force.' It describes the constant movement of vital energy through the body, mind, and spirit. Tibetan medicine, tantra, yoga, and Ayurveda principles base their healing techniques around the concept of Prana. Although the practices created to heal and maintain the properties of Prana are different from the Chinese Qi and the Japanese Ki, they all construct the value of these healing principles around the concept of life force.

Consider the concept of "light," or as the Christian philosophies and religions call it, the "Holy Spirit." Some might understand Christianity to display the idea of a Holy

Spirit as something available only to God, Christ, and the most devout followers of this religion who experience angelic miracles during their life on Earth. The concepts of Ki, Qi, and Prana all seem to make this source of energy available to everyone through their separate and different teachings, explaining that this Universal Life Force is a part of everyone and must be treated as such.

What you can understand about all of these different terms and cultural ideas is that they all point directly to the same idea: life force. The practice of Reiki is a clear, simple, and healing experience that allows you to channel life force for the purpose of healing. The practice of Reiki may be historically newer than some of the other cultural practices, but it delivers the same material through the energy centers of the body for awakening, enlightenment, truth, and healing.

## Mind, Body, Spirit, Wholeness

Once you can understand and accept the reality of our Universal Life Force, you can begin to see and comprehend that everything and everyone is a whole. You cannot heal only the physical self without healing the spirit or the mind. The greatest balance in all things comes with the completion of the cycle of three: mind, body, and spirit.

All of the information in this book so far has been written to address the main concepts and origins of Reiki. The central theme of what has been discussed is 'life force.' This concept is the umbrella that contains your mind, body, and spirit. One does not thrive or function well when another one is out of balance.

The effort of any healing practice that has been mentioned is to align these three components so that they operate harmonically. Each chakra is a spiritual center that has a direct effect on specific thoughts and emotions, as well as specific body functions and organ systems. One simply doesn't work without the other, and they should not be seen separately. They are life force.

As you progress forward through these pages and expand or refresh your knowledge of Reiki, remember that when you channel its energy, you are connecting to the universal properties that are already a part of you. The attunement to Reiki is to show you that you have the capability of healing and wholeness of all parts of you. Only when they are treated separately do you remain imbalanced.

For healing to occur on the whole system, the whole system must be acknowledged. Your mind, body, and spirit are one whole energy that is waiting to be loved, healed, nourished, revitalized, and restored to its original oneness.

The next parts of the book will be more in-depth training and understanding about the purpose of each degree and what quality of healing you may expect to experience.

# Part 2: The First Degree

# Chapter 3: Purpose of the First Degree

Your training starts here. You may have received a Reiki treatment once or twice and were amazed by the notable impact of how it can change your life experience. Often, once people are attuned to Reiki, they want to explore more deeply and connect to all of the possibilities available through energy healing.

The First Degree begins the journey and maintains an important point: before you help heal others, you must first heal yourself. The purpose of the First Degree is to attune you to Reiki so that you are an open channel to receive and transmit energy through your hands. Then, you are shown how you can heal yourself and eventually apply the same principles to another individual.

## Attunements

Attunements of the First Degree are typically performed on a person in a session or workshop with a practitioner of Reiki or a Master. It is the initiation that opens your physical body to the healing energy.

Traditional Japanese Reiki practices utilize four attunements, but the current Western practice has compiled it into one attunement. Every attunement utilizes a series of symbols: Japanese characters that are drawn in the air around the aura of the person receiving the attunement.

The practitioner uses their hand like a paintbrush, carving symbols energetically in the space around the receiver as an act of cleansing and opening. This initiation will transmit Reiki energy through the practitioner's hands into the receiver of the attunement. The difference between this experience and a regular Reiki session that you give or receive are the symbols.

The symbols speak and draw the attention and focus of attuning the person to become aligned with this energy to use for healing. In order to become attuned, you must seek a practitioner to initiate you with the first-degree attunement. Then, you will have access to Reiki energy forever; it does not close or require re-attunement.

## Self-Healing

The intention of Reiki Level One surrounds healing of the self. What this means is that once you are attuned to Reiki, you must practice this energetic healing through your own hands on your own body. Many people may have the urge to hurry the process by going forward to heal others, but this is not advised.

If you want to be truly helpful to others, you must first help yourself. In Part 1, you learned some history and background of Reiki, which is common as part of Level One Reiki training. You also discovered information about the chakras and auras, which are directly linked to your overall healing process. As you become attuned to the First Degree, your body will likely react and begin the healing process through your energy centers. This purging of toxins, outdated beliefs, emotional imbalance, and early life traumas will manifest in a variety of ways. It can be stronger for some and very subtle for others.

You may feel body aches, soreness, headaches, exhaustion, and emotional releases such as uncontrollable tears or laughter. It is different for everyone because everyone is different. When these symptoms arise, if they do, it is the perfect opportunity to utilize Reiki to help restore vitality to the areas that are going through healing and release as a result of level one attunement.

You now have the ability to start your self-healing journey. Keep a journal of your physical and emotional symptoms, as well as any thoughts that may arise. All of these experiences are there for healing through Reiki. Keeping a record of your self-healing process may be useful as you begin to work with others.

This time in your life will be very memorable. It is the beginning of a life-long relationship with Reiki and having the ability to heal yourself. It is always good to seek medical advice for many conditions; however, Reiki can be used to assist any medical treatments you may have and help improve your recovery and healing time for any procedures.

To begin your self-healing journey, you will learn the hand positions that you will use on yourself. You will use these same hand positions on other people or whomever you choose to work with, be it animal, vegetable, or mineral.

# Chapter 4: Hand Positions

The first degree hand positions are your tool for channeling and moving Reiki through your own or someone else's being. Become familiar with these positions because they are the bread and butter of practicing Reiki on anyone.

There is no right or wrong way to treat yourself. Reiki works so that, once you are attuned, it will naturally flow to where it is needed. If, however, you have chronic or acute conditions, you will want to draw focus to these areas.

Every time you treat yourself, use a full self-treatment. This means using every hand position in order. After you feel you have mastered the hand positions, you may feel ready to start using your intuition as a guide.

Each hand position should be maintained for 3 to 5 minutes. However, use your intuition to guide you. In most positions, your hands will be loosely or gently cupped to support and contain the flow of Reiki. Try to make hand positions slide and flow from one position to the next if you can. You can lay down to begin if you want. For position 12 you will need to be seated in a chair or on the floor.

Find a space where you will not be disturbed for your entire treatment. If you like, play some soothing music to help you engage with your spiritual energy.

### *Hand Position 1:*

Loosely cup your hands and gently place them over your eyes, cheekbones, and forehead. This placement connects to your third eye. Hold for 3 to 5 minutes.

This position helps with: stress; head issues like, colds, sinus issues, allergies, and asthma; connecting to and healing pituitary and pineal glands and cerebral nerves.

### *Hand Position 2:*

Place your hands on the top of your head so that your fingertips are pointing toward each other and your elbows are relaxed and pointed away from your body. This placement connects to your crown chakra and where Reiki flows through for channeling. Hold for 3 to 5 minutes.

This position helps with: eye issues, headaches, migraines, stress, bladder and digestive disorders, multiple sclerosis, flatulence, and emotional problems.

### *Hand Position 3:*

Place hands on either side of your head with your palms covering your temples, loosely cupped, fingers curving toward the top of your head, elbows out to the side. Hold for 3 to 5 minutes.

This position helps with: tinnitus, inner ear problems, hearing issues, balance, vertigo, colds and flu, and balance between the right and left brain.

### *Hand Position 4:*

Place gently cupped hands on the back of the head on the occipital ridge. (*The occipital ridge is at the base of the skull, just before your neck*). Your fingers should be touching. Hold for 3 to 5 minutes.

This position helps with: eye problems, headaches, stress, stroke, fears and phobias, sinuses, hay fever, shock, depression, and digestive disorders.

### *Hand Position 5:*

From Position 4, slide hands down the neck to its base, where the neck and shoulders meet. Keep hands relaxed and loosely cupped. Hold for 3 to 5 minutes.

This position helps with: tight neck and shoulders, aches and pains, stress, shock, and spinal injury.

### *Hand Position 6:*

Slide hands forward to the front of the neck so the heels of your hands are touching in front of your throat, elbows in front of you, touching, or nearly touching. This position connects to your throat chakra. Hold for 3 to 5 minutes.

This position helps with: breathing, communication, voice or speech problems, bronchitis, flus and colds, self-expression, and anger. It also connects to the thyroid gland.

### *Hand Position 7:*

From the throat position, bring hands down to form a T-shape over the heart: the left hand over the heart, fingers pointing toward right shoulder; right hand slides down and curves slightly to the side so fingers are comfortably pointing up toward the chin, and the hand is positioned in front of the lower sternum. Make sure the hands are touching and not separated. (\**Regarding handedness, if it is more comfortable for you to reverse this so that your right hand is crossing your heart and your left hand is pointing up toward your chin, that's okay. Trust your comfort*). Hold for 3 to 5 minutes.

This position helps with: emotional matters, lung and breathing issues, angina, weight problems, and immune and lymph system. It also connects to the thyroid and thymus glands.

***Hand Position 8:***

Position hands on the pectoral muscles, just above the nipples, palms gently cupped. Fingers should be pointing toward each other, elbows to the side. Hold for 3 to 5 minutes.

This position helps with: *see Hand Position 11*.

***Hand Position 9:***

From Position 8, move hands down the torso so that they are positioned just below the rib cage. This position connects to the solar plexus chakra. Hold for 3 to 5 minutes.

This position helps with: *see Hand Position 11*.

***Hand Position 10:***

From Position 9, slide hands slowly and gently to just above the hip bones. This position connects to the sacral chakra. Hold for 3 to 5 minutes.

This position helps with: *see Hand Position 11*.

***Hand Position 11:***

From Position 10, slide your hands down to the very bottom of your hips where they connect with the top of your thighs. Point your fingers inward to form a triangle or V-shape with the sides of your pointer fingers and thumbs. This position connects to the root chakra. Hold for 3 to 5 minutes.

This position helps with: all major organs and gland systems, infections, disease, intestines and stomach, reproductive organs, anger, and all emotions.

***Hand Position 12:***

From a seated position, place your hands over the front of the knees. Hold for 3 to 5 minutes.

This position helps with: *see Hand Position 13*.

***Hand Position 13:***

From Position 12, slide hands under to the back of your knees so that your hands are gently cupping here. Hold for 3 to 5 minutes.

This position helps with: pain in the legs, circulation, stiff or sore knees, knee injury, and varicose veins.

*\*Note: The next few positions will work on your back side. Please work with your comfort level and flexibility. Keep the body relaxed as you remain in a seated position.*

***Hand Position 14:***

Begin with your hands on your shoulders, elbows directly out to the side. Hands should be gently cupped. Hold for 3 to 5 minutes.

This position helps with: *see Hand Position 17*.

***Hand Position 15:***

From Position 14, bring your hands around to your back, as high as they can go with your palms facing your back, hands gently cupped and relaxed. Do not over-extend if you have limited flexibility. Work from a lower position and direct energy up the back as needed. Try to get your hands close enough so that your fingers touch. This position should be in line with and connect to the solar plexus chakra, like Hand Position 9. Hold for 3 to 5 minutes.

This position helps with: *see Hand Position 17*.

***Hand Position 16:***

From Position 15, slide the hands slowly and gently down to the lower back, just above the top of the hips. Finger tips remain touching. This position connects with your sacral chakra. Hold for 3 to 5 minutes.

This position helps with: *see Hand Position 17.

### *Hand Position 17:*

From Position 16, slide hands down to form a V-shape or triangle, like Hand Position 11. Your hands should be covering your sacral bone and tail bone. This position connects to the root chakra. Hold for 3 to 5 minutes.

This position helps with: the major organ and gland systems, disease, infections, back and spinal issues and discomforts, and stress.

### *Hand Position 18:*

You should already be seated, but if you are in a chair, try sitting on the ground in the lotus position: bottom on the floor, soles of the feet touching each other, knees pointed out to the side. Hold both feet with your hands so that the palms of your hands are touching the top of your feet. Hold for 3 to 5 minutes.

*Modification: If it is uncomfortable for you to sit in this position, you can sit with your legs crossed and perform 3 to 5 minutes of Reiki on each foot, one at a time. Use both hands to cup the sole and top of your foot, and then switch to the other.*

This position helps with: all major organ and gland systems, leg pain and circulation issues, varicose veins, and grounding to the Earth. It heals Reflexology points.

## Ending a Self-Treatment

At the end of your treatment, you can take a moment to just sit and feel the difference in your body. Use another 3 to 5 minutes to meditate on your new feelings or what emotions or sensations might have come up during your session with yourself. When you feel ready to move forward in the day, be sure to drink some purified water after your treatment to help your body cleanse the toxins that were accessed for release and purging.

Throughout the day, notice any symptoms, emotions, side-effects, and physical feelings awakened during your session. If it is helpful, note it in your healing journal so that you can keep track of the healing journey as you progress.

One major thing to keep in mind: if your body, mind, or spirit wants you to rest after a session, it is important to do so. You may need time to lay down and let your whole being process the energetic healing that occurred. Let yourself recover. Some experiences may feel more intense than others.

These hand positions will be used in every Reiki healing you do. They don't change. When you are channeling Reiki to help others, your stance may change, and the way you hold your hands in relation to their body may alter slightly, but these positions are the basic tools for performing a Reiki treatment on yourself and anything else.

Commit it to your mind like a dance that you meditate through, with Reiki as your guide.

## Healing Common Ailments

In the First Degree, the main practice is to heal the self to gain a deeper understanding of Reiki and how it flows through you. You will get to experience first-hand how it feels, how long it takes, what the side-effects might be, and how you will feel once you have healed various ailments and issues.

Many of us walk through life with common ailments that we complain about but learn to live with and even ignore. Coping with chronic pain, stress, headaches, allergies, sleep problems, worry, and doubt leaves us feeling depleted every day of our life force energy. Sometimes, people will end up taking over-the-counter medications that do nothing to treat the whole problem.

Reiki is an excellent tool for healing common ailments. You don't need to be a doctor of medicine to heal through Reiki. All you need is to allow the energy to channel through your hands and into your body. Reiki goes where it is needed.

*Note of Caution: If you are concerned about your health, see a medical professional. Reiki does not prescribe or diagnose.*

Follow your intuition about staying in certain areas. If you have chronic neck and shoulder pain, stay holding hand positions in these areas until you feel a noticeable shift. There isn't a time limit, and you will notice when it is time for the next hand position. Some areas may need more focused attention than others. Let your intuition tell you what you need. When you are attuned to Reiki, you are attuned to your intuition, and with practice, you will be able to easily feel what needs the most focus and for how long.

# Chapter 5: Practice Healing Others

Learning to channel Reiki is exciting! You are open to the Universal Life Force, have healed yourself, and truly begun to understand what it means to live a whole, healthy, and connected life. Knowing what it means and how it can help you naturally encourages a wish to help others. If you have the knowledge and ability to channel healing, why wouldn't you?

For some, the act of self-healing is enough for engaging in a new, healthy lifestyle and transformation. For many, the intention is to share this technique to aid others in following their truth and reconnecting to their power to heal themselves. This a remarkable way to connect to all things: healing others leads to community and unconditional love and healing.

As we collectively embrace our Universal Life Force, we invite healing not just for ourselves or for a small group, but for all living things across the globe.

After you become attuned in the First Degree, you will spend three weeks to three months holding space for your own healing journey. Listen to your intuition for how long you spend in this phase. You may feel ready sooner than three weeks, and you may need longer than three months—every person is different and responds differently to Reiki. You will likely know when you are truly ready to bring Reiki to another living person, plant, or animal.

## Preparing to Treat Others

Before you begin to channel Reiki to help others, it is important to create the right setting, time, and space. An appropriate environment to offer Reiki treatments will be clean, light, and peaceful, free of distractions and have a feeling of safety. It should be a comfortable temperature and if soothing music is desired, having a way to include that in the experience is best organized prior to treatment. A strong recommendation is to have a box of tissues handy. Sometimes, Reiki can have an effect that causes emotional release, and being prepared for that will help the person receiving feel safe to express and purge these emotions.

If you are interested in having a professional Reiki space, you can get more detailed with the room design and comfort. Bring in some plants and crystals to add positive energy to the space. Offer aromatherapy and essential oils as long as the client does not react strongly to scents.

It is recommended that you acquire a therapeutic table or massage table if you want to offer Reiki professionally. This allows your client to fully relax, and by allowing them to lie down, you have greater access to the areas that need treatment. A table like this will assist the success and comfort of your practice. You will need sheets, blankets (in case the client gets cold), and pillows.

If you are interested in a more casual practice at first and are not ready to set up a Reiki healing space yet, you can accommodate clients by having them sit upright in a chair or have a comfortable way for them to lie down. You can find stretch mats for the ground and perform entire sessions on the floor, as long as your body is comfortable channeling in this way.

Before you begin a Reiki treatment to help someone, it is important for both the giver and receiver to remove all pieces of jewelry and tight clothing or accessories (this also goes for self-practice). It is important that each person feel relaxed. Metal jewelry can react to the energy of Reiki and have an impact on the strength of energy being channeled into the client. Remove belts, ties, shoes, and anything else that might feel uncomfortable while you are performing the treatment.

When you offer treatment to someone, give them that information ahead of time. Let them know when they come for their Reiki session that they need to wear loose or comfortable clothing and leave off all jewelry and accessories. That way, they will arrive prepared.

It is necessary to make sure you practice good hygiene before working on others. Be cleaned and washed, avoiding strong soaps, perfumes, and lotions. Be sure you have fresh breath. Wash your hands before you perform a treatment, making sure your fingernails are clean. Make sure to also wash your hands after treatment.

Prior to offering Reiki, it is necessary to avoid drugs or alcohol for at least 24 hours. Alcohol will dissipate the energy and cloud your channel for Reiki. If you want to provide your client or the person receiving the Reiki with the clearest healing, then you must be prepared to be a channel, free of toxins that can impede the flow of Reiki.

If you are not planning on professionally offering Reiki treatments and are only looking to aid your friends, family, and pets, then you can modify your approach to treatment. You may not need a professional set up to help the people in your life and your immediate circle of acquaintances. It is still a good idea to practice the basics of a professional approach even when working with close relations:

- Create a safe, warm, and comfortable environment.
- Eliminate distractions, like cell phones, TV, or interruptions by other people.
- Avoid alcohol for at least 24 hours.
- Practice good hygiene before and after treatment.
- Be prepared for emotional release with a box of tissues.

Now that you have made all of the preparations, you can begin a Reiki treatment. You are attuned to Reiki and have practiced all of the hand positions on yourself for three weeks to three months and feel prepared to channel Reiki into another for healing. You will need to connect yourself to the experience with an invocation.

## Invocation

It is important to remember that as a Reiki practitioner, you are not healing anyone. People receive Reiki through you and they are healing themselves. You are the conduit or channel that provides them with the energy, and they are the ones doing the healing.

When you internally invoke Reiki before beginning with your client, you are giving up any claims to healing power; you are acknowledging that you are a channel and that is all. The invocation helps you to center and ground in that truth and the principles of Reiki before you open up the healing channel for Reiki to come through you into your client's auric field and chakras.

Your invocation should be personal to you. It can refer or call upon your Reiki teacher or Master who attuned you, as well as the Masters before them like Usui, Hayashi, Takata, etc. As long as it connects to you, your personal beliefs, and your intuition, then it will be exactly what you need to be a clear channel for Reiki.

You can recite your invocation in your head prior to the treatment, standing at the head of the table where the client's head would be laying or standing behind them if they are seated in a chair.

Place your hands in front of your heart in a prayer position, eyes closed or open, depending on your preference, and invoke the healing energy of Reiki.

Here is an example invocation to give you an idea of how it might look:

"I call upon Reiki, the Universal Life Force, angelic beings, and masters who have healed with Reiki before, including (*insert master or teacher's name here*), and all the Reiki Masters from the past, present, and future to draw near and participate in this healing session. I ask for the wisdom and healing power of Reiki to permit me to be a channel of unconditional love and healing energy on behalf of (*insert client's name*). May the infinite wisdom of Reiki travel where it needs to go mostly for the higher good of (*insert client's name*). May we all be empowered by Divine love and Universal Life Force."

Once you have spoken your invocation, you are connected to Reiki and the energy of the space and moment. You can now be a channel of Reiki and preform a healing treatment.

## The Treatment Experience

The treatment session for anyone you channel Reiki for will be similar to a treatment that you give yourself. The hand positions are alike. However, the length of time you maintain a hand position depends on the client, their ailments, and how the energy is flowing. Use your intuition and let it guide you. Keep a clock nearby that can help you with the timing at first, but as you develop and trust your intuition, you won't need to keep track of minutes.

Some things to keep in mind as you prepare to treat someone:

- Use your intuition.

- Remember the Reiki Principles: what they mean and how they impact our lives.
- You do not need a thorough knowledge of anatomy to provide this experience.
- The client draws Reiki through you; you are not healing them.
- Reiki does the work, not you. Ego is left at the door.
- Forget the symptoms and treat the whole person.
- Pay attention to any non-verbal communication coming from the receiver's body. Awareness of their experience can help guide you. Listen to their body with your hands.
- Your hands may feel hot and may also feel cold.
- Don't expect dramatic effects or reactions with every person. Even when the effects aren't obvious, Reiki is still doing the healing work.
- Trust yourself; trust Reiki.

## Step 1: Reiki Intake Process

Before you give a Reiki treatment to anyone, whether it is a friend, family member, or client, you must perform an intake to assess any possible contraindications. A contraindication is a word that describes an acute or chronic problem that may be negatively affected by Reiki treatment. There are officially no known contraindications for using Reiki; however, there are two possibilities to be aware of that have come up in recent times:

- *Pacemakers*: According to some experiences, Reiki can disrupt or alter the rhythm of a pacemaker, requiring the person with it to have issues and a need to see their cardiologist to reset the rhythm.
- *Diabetes*: If someone is suffering from diabetes and taking insulin, Reiki can reduce the amount of insulin required. This is a good thing as it may help heal a person's need for insulin and improve their diabetic condition, but they must be

prepared to monitor and check their insulin levels daily if they are wanting Reiki treatments.

Once you have established an understanding with the client about these two factors, it is a good practice to communicate with them prior to treatment about what they can expect from the experience and what side effects may occur.

Explaining the process in simple terms will comfort them about their experience. Letting them know that they may have natural reactions to the energy healing will also provide comfort. Explain that they may or may not:

- Feel sensations of hot or cold
- See colors or light
- Have flashes of past lives
- Involuntary movements in their body
- Fall asleep
- Feel itchiness
- Have an emotional reaction or response
- Feel a gurgling stomach
- Experience memory flashbacks
- Feel a sensation of pins and needles
- Sense the hands of the Reiki practitioner, even though they are not in physical contact with the body

Let them know that it is also normal to feel none of the things or to feel it so subtly that it is hardly noticeable.

Approaching the client in this manner will help them feel prepared for a healing experience.

## Step 2: Cleanse and Harmonize the Aura

Now that you have an understanding about the auras, you can picture in your head the layers of energy outside of the body with which you will be working. The aura cleansing process is an excellent way to build rapport with your client and their energy. It is the first step to bringing Reiki to the client for healing. It is almost like making an introduction or shaking hands with someone's energy field.

With the client lying face up on the table, you will cleanse the aura three times. Place your hands six inches above the client's body and run your hands, slow and smooth, from their head to their feet.

When you perform this action, you are also 'feeling out' potential areas where there may be blockages or areas of focus for the Reiki treatment. These areas may feel hot, cold, or stuck. Use your intuition to paint a mental map of these places. Working with your eyes closed during an aura cleanse can help you feel and 'see' the energy more clearly.

Be sure to cleanse the aura three times before you progress into the treatment. A full Reiki treatment on a client should last at least an hour and may take up to 90 minutes, depending on the person and their energy needs.

You are now ready to channel Reiki through your hands and into the client.

## Hand Positions for Treating Others

Before you begin the treatment, be sure to wash and dry your hands thoroughly. Your full body treatment should last for 60 to 90 minutes without interruption.

The client should begin the treatment facing up (supine) on the table. At a certain point in the session, you will have them gently roll over onto their stomach (prone).

Begin with your invocation, followed by an aura cleansing.

Remember, for each position you will need to hold it at least 3 to 5 minutes. The more experienced you become, the better you can gauge this timing for each individual.

Avoid areas of the body with severe skin burns. Also, make sure that you are respecting the private areas of the client, assuring that as you pass over breasts and genitals, your hands are not touching them, but hovering above the body. These areas are not to be touched under any circumstances during a Reiki session.

In general, when giving Reiki treatment to a person, you don't actually have to touch their bodies. Some people want the healing experience, but do not want to be touched. You can give effective treatment to anyone without making physical contact. In fact, some Masters teach Reiki in this way.

Like with your personal Reiki treatments, your hands should be gently cupped with fingers closed like the Queen of England waving to her royal subjects.

These hand positions are only a guide. They structure the session with your client, but as you practice Reiki more, you will find yourself open to your intuition and feel guided by the energy exactly where you need to go and for how long.

*Note: You may work from a seated position at the head of the client table from Hand Positions 1 through 6. If you feel it will disturb your energy flow to move from seated to standing, then work from a standing position with your table at a level that won't hurt your back. You can play around with body mechanics more as you become more practiced in offering Reiki.*

### Hand Position 1:

Standing at the head of the table where the client's head is positioned, cup your hands over the client's eyes, cheekbones, and forehead. Fingers will be pointing toward their navel. Hold for 3 to 5 minutes.

### Hand Position 2:

From Position 1, bring your hands to the crown of the head like you are smoothing their hair back from their forehead. Hold for 3 to 5 minutes.

*Hand Position 3:*

Bring your cupped hands around to the side of the head with your palms covering their temples. You may also slightly cover their ears. Hold for 3 to 5 minutes.

*Hand Position 4:*

To get from Position 3 to 4, you will gently shift the head to one side to get your hands under their head to their occipital ridge or the base of the skull. Shift the head one direction and place one hand under the head. Then, with your hand under the head, help to shift their head in the opposite direction where you can then place your other hand. Both hands should then be cradling the base of the skull. Hold for 3 to 5 minutes.

*Hand Position 5:*

From Position 4, you will repeat the same process you used to place your hands under their head. Gently rock their head to one side to remove, freeing one hand to gently rock it the other direction, then freeing the second hand. You can then move to Position 5, placing your cupped hands along the jawbone and around the front of the neck so that your hands are covering their throat. Fingertips should be touching under the chin. Hold for 3 to 5 minutes.

*Hand Position 6:*

Bring your hands down to the client's shoulders. Hold for 3 to 5 minutes.

*Hand Position 7:*

Like the Hand Position 7 for self-care, you will be forming a T-shape over the client's heart chakra, over the sternum and lower ribs. You will need to position your body at this point so that you are standing at the side of the table. Place one hand across the heart above the nipple line and the other hand below it, fingers pointing up toward the chin, creating the T-shape. Hold for 3 to 5 minutes.

*Hand Position 8:*

From Position 7, you will move the hands down to the bottom of the rib cage so that one hand is on either side of the ribs. All your fingers should be pointing in the same direction away from your own body. Hold for 3 to 5 minutes.

*Hand Position 9:*

Move your hands from Position 8 down to the area just below the navel, at the sacral chakra level. Maintain your hand position from Position 8. Hold for 3 to 5 minutes.

*Hand Position 10:*

Shift your hands down further along the body to create the V-shape at the bottom of the hips and top of the thighs like you did in the Hand Position 9 for self-care. This will be the closest to the root chakra. Hold for 3 to 5 minutes.

*Hand Position 11:*

Follow the line of the legs down to the top of the knees and cup your hands gently, one over each knee. Hold for 3 to 5 minutes.

*Hand Position 12:*

Continue down the leg from the knees so that you are standing at the foot of the table, instead of the side. Place one cupped hand over the top of each foot. Hold for 3 to 5 minutes.

*Hand Position 13:*

Before you can begin Hand Position 13, you will need to ask your client to turn over into the prone position so that their stomach is on the table. Many therapeutic tables come with face cradles to avoid having to turn the neck and head to one side for too long. If this is not an option for you, help the client feel comfortable with pillows. They may have fallen asleep, and you will need to gently wake them and help them carefully shift into the face-down position.

For Position 13, begin at the side of the table, and place one hand over each shoulder blade. Hold for 3 to 5 minutes.

## Hand Position 14:

Slowly glide your cupped hands down the back to the area of the middle back or middle rib cage. Hold for 3 to 5 minutes.

## Hand Position 15:

Glide your hands down a little further down the back to the lower ribs and lower back region. On the front of the body, this would be the area just below the navel. Hold for 3 to 5 minutes.

## Hand Position 16:

Move the hands further down to the lowest part of the back where the top of the hips are at the iliac crests. Hold for 3 to 5 minutes.

## Hand Position 17:

Move your hands to the base of the spine to form the T-shape like you did in Position 7, placing one hand across the sacrum, fingers pointing away from you and the other hand making the base of the T, fingers pointing toward the client's head. Hold for 3 to 5 minutes.

## Hand Position 18:

Move your hands down the legs to the back of the knees and cup hands gently here. Hold for 3 to 5 minutes.

## Hand Position 19:

Finally, travel down the legs and stand, once again, at the foot of the table, cupping your hands over the soles of the feet. Hold for 3 to 5 minutes.

## Hand Position 20:

Once all positions have been performed, walk back to the side of the table and place one cupped hand over the crown chakra and one over the base of the spine. Hold for at least 3 to 5 minutes. This final position will balance the energy of the recipient and bring closure to the treatment.

*Aura Cleanse*

Before you end, comb your client's aura as you did at the beginning of the session, doing it three times. Each time you do it, you will touch the floor at the end to bring grounding and earth energy to yourself and the client.

The first stroke should be firm from head to feet followed by touching the ground. Then, do a light stroke from head to feet and touch the ground. Then, the lightest stroke above the body in the auric field ending with a touch to the floor.

Gently let your client know that the session has ended. They may have fallen asleep. Give them a moment to wake up and sit up while you get them a glass of water. Always offer water to your client after the session to refresh them and help them purge any toxins released during treatment.

## Express Reiki Treatment

There are some situations that require treatment for a shorter duration. You may need to help someone or yourself in a pinch due to an emergency or lack of time. Of course, this is possible, though it may not have as intense an effect as a full treatment.

Quick Reiki sessions are still valuable in their healing effects and should be learned for those moments when they are needed.

This usually occurs with the client seated in a chair or massage chair. You will also need a chair for yourself. Your focus will mainly be on the chakra points. This treatment should last 15 to 30 minutes.

*Hand Position 1:*

Begin standing behind your client with one hand cupped over each shoulder. Say your invocation and establish an energetic connection with your client. Hold for as long as it takes to say the invocation to yourself or longer if you feel it is necessary.

*Hand Position 2:*

Remain standing behind the client and place your hands cupped over the crown chakra. Hold for 3 to 5 minutes.

*Hand Position 3:*

Move to the side of the client and seat yourself in a chair for comfort (you will remain seated in the chair through Hand Position 7). Place one hand over the brow chakra and one hand over the occipital ridge (one in front, one in back). Hold for 3 to 5 minutes.

*Hand Position 4:*

Place one hand over the front of the throat, covering the throat chakra, and the other over the back of the neck. Hold for 3 to 5 minutes.

*Hand Position 5:*

Place one hand over the heart chakra, above the nipple line, and one hand over the back between the shoulder blades. Hold for 3 to 5 minutes.

*Hand Position 6:*

Place one hand cupped over the solar plexus chakra, just above the navel, and the other hand over the back of the spine, parallel to your hand in front. Hold for 3 to 5 minutes.

*Hand Position 7:*

Place one hand over the sacral chakra, just below the navel, and one hand over the lower back parallel to your hand in front. Hold for 3 to 5 minutes.

*Hand Position 8:*

Position yourself in front of the client (you may wish to bring your chair to the front or you can kneel). Place one hand over each knee. Hold for 3 to 5 minutes.

*Hand Position 9:*

Kneel in front of the client, if you are not already, and place one cupped hand over the top of each foot. Hold for 3 to 5 minutes.

*Finishing Treatment*

To end the express treatment, comb the aura three times like you would in a full treatment. Wash your hands and offer water to the client to help them ground.

You can offer this treatment to anyone who feels rushed for time but would benefit from Reiki. A little Reiki is better than no Reiki at all.

# Chapter 6: Other Applications with Reiki in the First Degree

### Solfeggio Frequencies

The Solfeggio Frequencies were discovered ages ago almost by accident. The idea was original, but the frequencies themselves have been a throbbing heartbeat of our Universe since the dawn of its birth.

Simply put, they are sound waves measured in hertz. Originally, St. John the Baptist had written hymns that followed a certain scale of sound used for spiritual incantation. There wasn't specific rhyme or reason to it; it was merely the sound of "God." Later, a Benedictine Monk by the name of Guido d'Arezzo (991 A.D.-1,050 A.D.) created the Solfeggio scale which was used in the church to help the singers learn the chants with greater ease.

The most notable scale that most us know is the 7-note scale taught in all music classes: *Do Re Mi Fa So La Ti.*

The Solfeggio scale has six notes: *Ut Re Mi Fa Sol La*

Sometime in the mid-1970s in America, an herbalist named Joseph Puleo was studying the scale and discovered six electromagnetic frequencies that corresponded to the Hymns of St. John. The frequencies were discovered through the Pythagorean Method, a mathematical equation that reduces numbers to their simplest form. For example:

$3{,}432 = 3 + 4 + 3 + 2 = 12 = 1 + 2 = 3$

Dr. Puleo and other researchers in sound therapy outlined the tones of the frequencies based on their Latin syllable association from the Solfeggio scale. The scale itself is a mathematical resonance that pierces the consciousness. Each frequency has the ability to change or alter energy in any living thing. The frequencies have been used since then to allow for deeper level healing of the mind, body, and soul.

Studies have been done to demonstrate the impact of sound on certain elements. Dr. Masaru Emoto, a Japanese author, wrote a book called *The Hidden Messages in Water* in which he demonstrates through experiment and photographs the impact of the sound wave on water. He froze the water to determine its shape after playing certain frequencies into the water. The results were astonishing. Classical music made gorgeous, geometric floral snowflake-like shapes, while dissonant, discordant sound or music created wobbly, inharmonious, blob-like shapes of distortion.

The experiment and other frequency healing trials have shown the immense impact of certain sounds on life.

The frequencies can be used to attain certain levels of healing and can be used in Reiki treatments. According to the Solfeggio Scale, they are:

- *Ut* - 346 Hz: turning grief into joy, liberation of guilt and fear
- *Re* - 417 Hz: undoing situations, facilitating change

- *Mi* - 528 Hz: transformation, miracles, repairing DNA
- *Fa* - 639 Hz: relationships, connections, spiritual family
- *Sol* - 741 Hz: expression, solutions, solving problems, cleansing
- *La* - 852 Hz: returning to spiritual order

Since the research of Dr. Puleo, there have been other experiments and tests performed to identify other healing frequencies. They are:

- 174 Hz: relief of pain
- 285 Hz: healing of the tissues
- 432 Hz: miracle tone
- 963 Hz: activation of pineal gland, opening of the third eye

Utilizing healing frequencies in Reiki therapies will bring more energetic balance, healing, harmony, and connection with the Universal Life Force. Let the sound heal with the Reiki.

## Reiki and Animals

As you know from your journey through learning Reiki, the applications are limitless. You can find a way to heal just about anything that is living. Our greatest companions can sometimes be non-human and furry, but they are of the same energetic force as humans. Cats and dogs have Reiki. Birds and fish have Reiki. Packs of wolves have Reiki.

What you can do with your knowledge of treating human beings in person or at a distance is apply it to working with animals. Whether they are domesticated or wild, they deserve a chance to heal, too. Animals benefit greatly from Reiki healing and you don't need to worry about getting verbal permission. Tell the animal in question what you wish to offer them. Be clear. They will let you know with their body language and attitude if they are interested or not. The rule of thumb in Reiki: use your intuition.

Apply the same principles, techniques, and treatment sessions you would to a human to any animal. You can project symbols from a distance or hold them in your lap and connect your channeled Reiki directly into them. You can also send healing to whole groups of wild animals or zoos if your heart is moved to do so. Again, the applications are limitless.

If you have a pet at home, practice on them. They'll always come back for more.

## Reiki in the Garden

What would happen if, rather than Miracle Grow you used Reiki Grow? Can you imagine how your garden would look? If you want to apply Reiki to your plants, indoor or outdoor, you can use your symbols and invoke activation of healing energy to anything that grows. Draw symbols in the soil where you plant your seeds. Put Reiki in your seeds. Charge the water you use before you water the garden. Bring Reiki to a whole field or forest. If you want to see Reiki at work, try an experiment:

1. Take a pack of seeds, any kind.
2. Divide the seeds into two groups.
3. Plant the first group in regular soil.
4. Take the second group and charge it with Reiki. Charge the soil before planting the seeds and the water before watering.
5. Place the two groups in pots or plots near each other.
6. Always use Reiki on group two. Never use Reiki on group one.
7. Sit back and enjoy.
8. After time, notice the difference in the seeds you planted from the same pack.

# Chapter 7: Conclusion of the First Degree

Your journey through the First Degree of Reiki is only the beginning. This first level attunes you to the Universal Life Force energy so that you may heal yourself and eventually aid others in healing themselves. It is in this First Degree that you are shown what may be hidden below the surface, what requires healing and balance, and what you can do to help yourself and someone else connect to your own healing power.

At the beginning of this journey, you will come across hidden feelings, emotions, and wounds. You may relive a trauma or even become acquainted with a past life lesson you are still learning in this current incarnation of your soul. You may have blocked memories resurface to be healed and released.

In whatever way it comes, the First Degree is how you come into healing your own soul. Once you begin to fully realize your universal gift, one shared by everyone, you will be ready to focus Reiki through your channels to help others awaken to their own healing magic.

You may decide that the first level is all you need to feel content and whole, in which case you would not need to progress further into the Second or Third Degree. Whatever your journey looks like, you now have the knowledge of how Reiki works, where it comes from, and how you are a channel for this energy and not a healer of others.

You will always have Reiki in you and around you whenever you need once you're attuned in the First Degree. How you decide to use this gift is up to you.

Once you find someone to give you your initial attunements, you will know how it feels to heal. The best way to understand Reiki is to feel it for yourself. If you have not yet been attuned by a Reiki practitioner or a Master, look in your area for ways to engage with the Reiki community. It is worldwide, and it is next door. Begin your journey today and heal yourself.

# Part 3: The Second Degree

# Chapter 8: Purpose of the Second Degree

Entrance into the Second Degree comes with time. You will have had some chances to heal yourself, practice on others, and become acquainted with the essence of Reiki energy. The Japanese word that is used in the Second Degree is *okuden*, which means "*deeper knowledge.*" If you were attending college, this would be like getting your masters, and the Third Degree would be your Ph.D.

The Second Degree is something you should only do when you feel ready. Working from the point of the first degree attunement, you will have strengthened your intuition. Use your intuition to help you decide if you are ready for the Second Degree. Some Western practices will give the first and second attunements in a one-weekend workshop. This can be intense, but if you have already done a good deal of healing work in the past and learned or used other therapies to cleanse your chakras or balance your energy, this may not feel as intense for you.

The purpose of the Second Degree is to go deeper into the knowledge and practice of Reiki, opening you to the more etheric fourth and fifth-dimensional possibilities using Reiki. What this means is that you will learn to use Reiki outside of one-on-one sessions with another person.

In the second level, you will learn the symbols. The symbols are a huge step in the practice of Reiki, and they open you to even greater abilities. Your ability and power strengthen by about four times of what it is in your first attunement. This increase is due to the symbols that you will be attuned to in your second level course. The symbols are generally kept secret and only passed from teacher/practitioner to student. For a long time, there was no known written knowledge of these symbols, however, many current masters and practitioners feel that offering this knowledge is acceptable, since Reiki is Universal energy.

You will still require a Reiki practitioner or master to attune you to the second level symbols to receive the benefits of using them.

This level will give greater balance to your seven chakras as you attune. You may go through an even deeper transformation of the self, sloughing off any remaining negativity, outdated mental programming, old behavior patterns that no longer serve the greater good, and purging emotions that lie in deeper layers. You will become more closely connected to your third eye and intuition, develop a more powerful connection to Reiki, and gain more confidence with allowing your intuition to guide you, rather than the traditional hand position movements. This stage is bonding with your own higher power and the power of the Divine. It is where you let go of skepticism and embrace belief and true knowing.

One of the biggest lessons of the Second Degree is distance healing. Distance healing allows you to provide Reiki treatment to anyone, anywhere, anytime. You will learn through the use of the symbols how to achieve this quality of channeling Reiki and sending across short or long, big or small distances. It is a way to connect to the past, present, and future.

You also receive understanding about how to use Reiki to channel healing to large groups, events, situations, and even cities or countries.

The Second Degree isn't a step; it's a quantum leap. Be prepared to take on more responsibility. Let your intuition tell you if you are ready to become a Second Degree Reiki practitioner.

# Chapter 9: Pillars of Reiki

The pillars of Reiki give form to the Five Principles of Reiki that you learned earlier in this book. The pillars present ideas and beliefs that are a foundation for understanding and living with Reiki, not just practicing it. The pillars are Gassho, Reiji Ho, and Chiryo.

### First Pillar: Gassho

*Gassho* (Japanese), pronounced "gash-show," means "two hands coming together." When you see images of monks in Buddhist temples with their palms pressed together in prayer, they are performing a Gassho. It is a fundamental mudra in Buddhism. A mudra is a gesture or body posture committed to the religious practice or elevated into the position held by deities.

The Gassho is a gesture that implies recognition of everyone and everything with humility. It is an expression of gratitude and respect for others no matter their background, religion, political affiliation, or skin color. It can be used to attain focus, and it creates a dynamic balance. Purely, it is an expression of oneness, totality, and congruence of being.

There are two main Gassho that you will learn here. You will find others as you continue in your journey through healing.

>1. **Formal Gassho:** This gesture is for rituals, ceremonies, and religious services. It expresses an attitude of reverence for higher realms and beings and the worship of the Divine. The hands are placed in prayer, palms together. They are away from the body with the fingertips aligned together and pointing 45 degrees out instead of up completely straight. They are pointing out and away to Universal Life Force. The hands are not overhead, but straight out from the heart chakra, elbows slightly bent.
>2. **Mu-Shin ("No Mind") Gassho:** This gesture is more of a greeting for anyone. The hands are close to the chest, unlike the formal Gassho, and the fingers are pointed up toward your chin. This is a simple way to say, 'I recognize you and have respect for you and all living things. We are one and the same.'

There are other forms of Gassho that are used by priests for special rights and ceremonies. Usui created a Gassho meditation for his Reiki students to use every day, morning, and night. This meditation will bring you relaxation, reduce stress, and connect you more deeply to Universal Life Force.

> - **Usui's Gassho Meditation** (5 to 20 minutes)
> **\*\*_Meditation for Stress Relief_**
>> 1. Sit down on the floor or on a cushion with legs comfortably crossed and eyes closed.
>> 2. Hold your hands in Mu-Shin.
>> 3. In your mind, focus your attention on the point of your hands where your middle fingers touch. Let go of everything else.

4. If thoughts wander, acknowledge your thought and simply return to the point of your touching middle fingers.

5. Repeat the Five Reiki Principles in your head or out loud if you are inclined. Do this anywhere from 5 to 20 minutes.

6. Repeat daily.

- **Namaste**

Another Gassho is the gesture represented in the concept '*Namaste*'. The gesture is accompanied by a head bow. It is a Sanskrit word that translates to '*I bow to you.*' It is the submitting of oneself to another with complete humility. In essence, it states:

*I honor the place in you in which the entire Universe dwells; the place of love, light, and peace. As I am in the place and as you are in that place, I honor that we are one. The spirit in me meets the spirit in you.*

This salutation between people also honors the duality of all things and how that duality or language of opposites creates the whole; one cannot exist without the other, as I cannot exist without you. You see these dualities in all things: sun/moon, man/woman, heaven/earth, thought/feeling, yin/yang.

This is an excellent gesture to perform anywhere in life, not just in your Reiki sessions. It is a sign of happiness expressed at the sight of seeing another. It is the shared ground between all people.

## Second Pillar: Reiji-Ho

*Reiji* means "indication of Reiki power," *Ho* means "methods." Reiji-Ho (pronounced ray-gee-hoe) is another form of Reiki meditation that is performed in three steps. It is a prayer method to connect to Reiki so that you can be guided by the energy, instead of simply performing a series of hand positions. It is also powerful to use this prayer in distance healing work.

*Step 1:*

Close your eyes and place your hands in Gassho. Connect with Reiki by asking in your mind three times for it to flow through you. As soon as you start to feel the Reiki energy rising and surging in you, move on to Step 2.

*Step 2:*

Raise your Gassho up from in front of your heart to your third eye. Ask for the recovery and health of the client on all levels should it be needed. Invite the Reiki to flow where it is needed. Ask the Reiki energy to guide your hands where the need is.

*Step 3:*

With your intentions made known through connection to Reiki, use your intuition to be guided. Feel the pull and tug of energy where you need to go. Let go of any attachments you may have to an outcome for the client. If at first you do not receive guidance, don't fret; it will come with time and practice. When you do not feel pulled toward any more areas that require treatment, your hands will be guided to stop.

Complete Reiji-Ho with Gassho.

*You can perform Reiji-Ho after your Invocation, although you may choose to perform this at another point in your healing session. Trust your intuition.*

## Third Pillar: Chiryo

The word *Chiryo* (pronounced chee-rye-oh) means "treatment." In this pillar, the practitioner places their dominant hand above the crown chakra of the receiver and here waits for an impulse or inspiration. This may require a few moments of focus in this hand placement, but once you feel an impulse, allow the hand to move wherever it needs or wants to go.

During the treatment, you will use your intuition in this way, giving free reign to the hands so that you can truly act as a channel for Reiki. Giving into the Reiki flow, your hands will automatically know where to travel. They are pulled to the painful areas and blockages and will remain there until these places are relieved through Reiki. Once you feel the energy dissipate, you allow your hands to flow to the next place.

Preparing for this pillar comes with practice of the others but can also be prepared for through the use of cleansing breath. Usui taught a breathing practice to help cleanse the spirit. Breath is considered the bridge between the body and consciousness. We are inhaling Reiki when we breathe in deeply; it clears the mind, body, and spirit.

- **Joshin Kokyuu Ho ("Breathing to Cleanse the Spirit"): Usui's Breath Meditation**

*Step 1:*

1. Sit on the floor, legs comfortably crossed and spine straight.
2. Inhale through the nose.
3. Imagine Reiki coming through your crown chakra into your body.
4. Hold awareness of that feeling and imagery for several moments.
5. Feel your body become enriched with Reiki.

*Step 2:*

1. Breath deep down into your tanden (area just below your navel).
2. Hold your breath in this area for a few moments and allow the breath to supply your body with vital energy.
3. Allow this energy to feel love and gentleness.
4. See the tanden energy spread throughout the whole body.

*Step 3:*

> 1. Exhale through your mouth and imagine that Reiki is flowing out of your mouth with your breath. See it coming out of your mouth, fingers, palms, toes, and soles.
> 
> 2. Feel yourself as a clear channel through this cleansing breath, allowing energy to flow into you through the cosmic inhale and out of you through the cosmic exhale.

*\*An advanced modification when you are feeling comfortable performing this breath meditation is to put your tongue on the roof of your mouth, touching the tip to the back of your top teeth as you inhale, and letting the tongue fall to the bottom of the mouth, touching the bottom teeth when you exhale.*

## Practicing Pillars of Reiki

As you progress through your Second Degree Reiki experience, you will begin to understand the pillars and principles and how incorporating them into your practice will bring you the energetic essence of healing and harmony that will keep you in the flow of Reiki.

Practicing Reiki will naturally call you to higher knowing and understanding. Bringing the pillars into your practice deepens and expands your intuition and your connection to the Universal Life Force.

# Chapter 10: The Sacred Reiki Symbols

The Reiki symbols are one of the most profoundly used tools in Reiki. If you wish to deepen your knowledge beyond the first level of knowing and understanding Reiki, then you will encounter the wisdom of the symbols created by Usui. His aim was to help explain to his students how to understand and connect more easily with Reiki. Originally, he taught Reiki without these symbols, but as his teaching evolved, so did his techniques. The symbols, whose meaning was originally found in the Sanskrit texts that Reiki energy was first described in, help to finely tune the Reiki as if you are tuning into a radio station and finding the placement of perfect reception.

The symbols are comprised of three main Japanese characters that have specific and special meaning in the Reiki practice. The fourth symbol is reserved for the student who wishes to become Master and is only received at the end of Master training.

Once you are attuned to these sacred symbols, they will be linked to your conscious and unconscious mind forever. For them to be properly embedded in your consciousness, you must already have been attuned in the Second Degree by a teacher or practitioner. These symbols will not work if you have not been attuned to the Second Degree.

## Why Learn and Use the Symbols?

The benefit of stretching your knowledge of Reiki to the next level is monumental. The increase in your energy and your ability to channel Reiki is four times stronger when you are attuned to the Second Degree as opposed to the first. Learning the symbols is an even greater enhancement to your experience channeling Reiki. Here are the benefits of learning and using the symbols:

- They help you connect more effectively to the energy.
- They are the keys that unlock the flow of energy, enhancing and amplifying it for stronger use.
- They harness focus and intuition.
- They bridge the gap between healer and recipient.
- They are powerfully beneficial in self-healing work as well as client work.
- The student will have four times higher vibration, allowing for stronger intuition and psychic ability.

You will discover more benefits as you learn to use these symbols. Remember, they are given to you in attunement of the second level of Reiki. You will learn what the symbols are and how to draw them in this book. Use it as a reference and guide as you work with your Master or practitioner.

*Note of Caution: You will likely go through a 21-day detoxification process when you are attuned to the symbols. Like in the first degree assimilation and re-balancing, your system will further purge what prevents the clear flow of Reiki energy through you.*

## Three Main Uses of Reiki Symbols

1. They increase focus with Universal Life Force for self-healing and healing of others.
2. There will be completion of full Reiki treatments in 15 minutes compared to the initial 60 to 90-minute sessions of the First Degree. Advanced practice and strengthened connection to the energy allows you to help more people in less time.
3. For distance healing, the Reiki symbols allow the ability to send healing energy across space and time; any person anywhere can receive treatment through a practitioner's use of these symbols.

The symbols have unlimited uses, and you are only limited by your imagination. The more you practice and explore, the more varied the applications you will discover.

## Preparing to Draw the Symbols

When you become attuned to the three Reiki symbols, you will commit them to your mind, body, and spirit; they will never leave you. They will become a part of your life as you draw them, picture them, see them, and send them again and again through your Reiki healing practice.

When drawing the symbols, your mind must be clear, positive, and light. You will likely have already called upon Reiki energy through invocation and any of the pillars before you begin to draw any of the symbols.

Understand that the symbols are living energy and are best visualized as such. Some will see them drawn in white light, but it will always depend on you and your connection with Reiki. There are six main ways you will draw the symbols during a Reiki healing session:

1. Imagine a bright, white symbol of light projected from the third eye onto the back of each of your hands as you rest them over the client.
2. Imagine a bright, white symbol of light drawn on the palms of your hands as you rest them over the client.
3. Draw a symbol on the roof of your mouth with your tongue, then project it onto the back of both your hands while they are resting over the client.
4. Draw a symbol on the roof of your mouth with your tongue, then project it onto both of your hands as you rest them over the client.
5. Draw the symbol on the palms of your hands using your index finger, then place your hand over the client.
6. Draw the symbol in the air with your finger in the direction you wish the Reiki to go.

As you draw each symbol, you will intone the name of the symbol three times, silently or aloud, to activate it. The symbol will not provide the power of the energy without the intonation.

*Modification for Drawing Symbols: In some cases, you may have questions about an issue that needs clarification or if you are working with someone across a distance. In this situation, you can write specific details, questions, names, etc. on the paper and then write the symbols on the paper to draw the healing energy.*

*Note: When you draw the Reiki symbols, you will always draw left to right and top to bottom. With each instruction for drawing a symbol, if the instructions ask you to draw a horizontal line, it will start at the left and be drawn across the page to the right. This is also true for starting a line at the top and finishing it at the bottom.*

## The First Symbol: Cho Ku Rei

Pronounced as cho-coo-ray, this is the most important symbol because it always activates the other symbols. It is sometimes called "the light switch" because it is the power symbol that brings light and energy to the others.

*Cho* – "to cut or remove illusion so one may see the whole"

*Ku* - "Penetrate (imagine a piercing sword)"

*Rei* - "Universal, present, and everywhere"

**How to Draw the First Symbol:**

> 1. Draw a horizontal line, left to right.
> 2. Beginning at the end of the first stroke, draw a longer vertical line going down.
> 3. At the bottom of the second stroke, begin drawing a spiral along all of the second line, making the spiral three rounds.

The symbol should look like a spiral with a long line through it and a short line at the top.

This symbol turns on or ignites the second degree energy. Without this symbol, you will only be channeling first degree energy. You can use this symbol by itself, but it will always be used to activate the other two symbols when you are using them.

**Example Uses of Cho Ku Rei:**

- Activates second degree energy
- Turns on and charges the other Reiki symbols
- Brings balance
- Acts as a protection on all levels
- Allows for whatever is needed in each situation
- Useful for cleansing energy in the home, car, workspace, crystals, etc.
- Can be used to charge and heal food and drink, plants, and animals.
- Bring energy, vitality, and healing to your career
- Useful when traveling on planes, trains, and automobiles
- Invisibly drawn under doormats, wallpaper, rugs, and furniture
- Sewn into clothing for protective energy

- Limitless potential, only limited by a lack of imagination

## The Second Symbol: Sei Heiki

Pronounced as say-high-key, this symbol is connected to the energy of healing emotional and mental blockages, pain, and imbalance. It also works to balance the right and left brain.

*Sei* – "birth, coming into existence"

*Heiki* – "equilibrium, balance"

**How to Draw the Second Symbol:**

> 1. Draw a zigzag in three parts: down, up, down. It should look like a lightning bolt (when drawn, it appears at a very subtle angle).
> 2. From the tail end of the lightning bolt, draw a short, vertical line straight down.
> 3. From the end of the third stroke, draw a wide semi-circle or backward C. *Strokes one through three should be one connected line.*
> 4. Starting where you began stroke 1, just to the right, draw another semi-circle or backward C so that it curves around the first three connected lines you drew.
> 5. Near the top of the curve in line 4, draw a small semi-circle or hump.
> 6. Repeat Step 5 just below the hump, making a second small hump. The small humps are close but not touching.

To activate this symbol, first draw the Cho Ku Rei symbol and intone the words Cho Ku Rei three times. This will activate the second symbol.

Then, draw Sei Heiki symbol, intoning the name three times.

Finally, intone three times and intone Cho Ku Rei again.

This is stacking the Reiki symbols to create more power activation and use.

This symbol is especially impactful if a client is suffering from serious emotional and mental blockages, addictions, unwanted habits, and weight problems. The stack of symbols will remove blockages and permit healing. It is like a sword cutting through all pain and negativity.

If you are using this stacked symbol to help in the healing of severe disease like cancer, leukemia, and AIDS, practice imagining thousands of Sei Reiki all over and around yourself or the other person.

Imagine drawing the symbol on your third eye and projecting it onto the third eye of your client. You may also draw the symbol over their head.

*Note of Caution: Take special care of your third eye in treatments with intense emotional/mental trauma. This symbol is a direct link to the mind of another person, and they will be connected to you through your third eye as well. Be prepared to protect and guard your thoughts as they might be picked up by your client. You may want to speak to the higher mind of the client to ask permission to go deep into their thoughts and emotions. You can also protect yourself with Reiki symbols intentionally in specific cases.*

**Example Uses of Sei Heiki:**

- Removes blockages and resistance in the body
- Relieves long-standing, deep issues
- Aids in healing addictions to alcohol, drugs, nicotine, and food
- Helps heal anorexia and bulimia
- Helps with relationship issues
- Cleanses issues of nervousness, fears, and phobias
- Helps heal anger, sorrow, depression, and toxic emotions
- Aids is healing grief from loss
- Helps those with head injuries or who have gone into a coma

- Calms negative spaces and atmospheres
- Helps improve memory and cognitive function
- Can enhance affirmations
- Improves intuition
- Calms arguments, discord, and conflict
- Heals negative and imbalanced communications
- Protection on every level
- Helping to find missing or lost things and protects from losing personal belongings
- Enhances creativity
- Useful for travelling

Never use these symbols to manipulate others. You will lose your gift of Reiki.

You can use the six main methods for drawing symbols mentioned earlier in this section. Any of them will work, but you will always draw the first symbol before activating the second.

## The Third Symbol: Hon Sha Ze Sho Nen

Pronounced as hon-sha-zee-show-nen, this is the symbol used for absent or distant healing and is used to transcend space and time. Like the second symbol, it is also activated by the Cho Ku Rei. When activated, Hon Sha Ze Sho Nen can send Reiki energy across any distance to any person, place, group, situation, part of the world, and even the past, present, and future.

It is the bridge between your past hurts and even your past lives that allows you to heal old pain from childhood and beyond. You can also send and promote healing to future situations or events. With this symbol, time and distance have no relevance.

It is a very powerful symbol and the most complicated to draw. The instructions for drawing this symbol will divide it accordingly between words, one word at a time. The symbol is meant to be written as one long, connected chain.

## How to Draw the Third Symbol:

*Hon* – "essence or cause"

>1. Draw a vertical line.
>2. Draw a line across that line like you are crossing a lowercase *t*.
>3. From the inside bottom corner of the cross, draw a line down to the left like you are drawing toward a corner.
>4. Do the same on the right side.
>5. Make a small horizontal stroke near the bottom part of the first stroke.

This first character, or kanji, is a symbol of a tree of transformation, death, desire resistance, etc. It is the first part of the third symbol.

*Sha* – "coming into existence"

>1. Draw a horizontal stroke (symbol of the land) just beneath the first character, Hon.
>2. From the end of line 6, draw a line down and to the left, curving slightly in a bow.
>3. From that bow or curve, about ¾ of the way down line 7, make a short, vertical line.
>4. From the starting point of line 8, the top of the line, draw a horizontal line out to the right and then a vertical line down in equal measure to the horizontal. It will look like you drew the corner half of a square for this line.
>5. Draw a short, horizontal line from left to right across the middle of line 8.

This second symbol connects to the first and begins the third. It means, "what is hidden is brought into being, bringing light to earth." It is a person who creates, an artist who turns color into image, or a potter who turns clay into pot.

*Ze* – "harmonizing appropriately"

>1. Draw a line downward, curving to the left.

2. Beginning at the same point as line 11, draw a line downward to the right. Together they make a curved, upside-down V-shape.

*Sho* – *"correctly or justly"*

1. Draw a horizontal line, just below that last character drawn.
2. From the center of that line, draw a vertical line down. It should look like a capital *T*.
3. Off to the left of the vertical line just drawn, but still under the umbrella of the first line, draw a short, little vertical line.
4. Midway down line 14, the long vertical line of the *T*, draw a short horizontal line like you are making an *F*.

This is a symbol of justice, correctness, and being/acting right.

*Nen* – "the heart of the thoughts, now"

1. Just below the last character drawn, make a small, horizontal line.
2. A little below that, draw another slightly longer horizontal line so that they are parallel, and the bottom line is slightly longer. At the end point of the horizontal line, draw a long, curved line down to the left like you are drawing a bowed 7.
3. To the right of the curved 7 tail, draw a semi-circle, or wide *C*.
4. Draw a smaller *c* inside the big *C*.
5. Draw a little backward *c* so that the top of it is next to the top of the big *C*, and the bottom of it curves into the middle of the little *c*. None of the semi-circles should be touching.

All of these characters, drawn stacked on top of each other, create the third symbol. It can be transferred from the self to the client in the same six ways detailed earlier in the chapter. Follow the same stacking principle you used in the second symbol to activate the third, however, you will use the first symbol, Cho Ku Rei, a total of three times.

Cho Ku Rei + Sei Heiki + Cho Ku Rei + Hon Sha Ze Sho Nen + Cho Ku Rei

This is the most powerful use of the symbols and the most powerful use of Reiki prior to becoming a Master.

**Example Uses of the Third Symbol:**

- Used for deep disease
- Helpful with deeply rooted issues, behaviors, and negative life patterns
- Can channel Reiki across distance and time
- Useful for large groups or organizations, even at a distance
- Can be used to channel healing towns, cities, and countries
- Works well with situations of disaster or crisis
- Can be sent to world leaders, politicians, and political organizations
- Excellent aid for interviews, meetings, and tests
- Medical exams, biopsies, and procedures
- Karmic, past life patterns, and issues
- Children while sleeping, resting, or ill
- Patients who cannot be touched because of risk of infection, such as burn victims
- Healing for the inner child
- Heals moments, periods, or traumas from the past and present
- Sends healing into future moments, situations, or events
- World Peace

The list is endless, and you can only be limited by a lack of imagination.

There are only three main Reiki symbols. Separately, they are powerful; together, they are potent. You must learn these symbols to practice Second Degree Reiki. Your second degree attunement will bring you into contact with these symbols. Once they are a part of your being, they can never leave or lose their power, unless you use them to manipulate others.

You must always gain permission to channel Reiki into another soul. Only then it can truly be of service. These symbols, along with the pillars and principles, are the bread and butter of Reiki. Know them well. Practice them daily. Eventually, you will get to a point where you have less of a need to reference them or see them to know what they are, what they look like, and what they mean.

The symbols are sacred and can be given to you when you are ready to receive your second degree attunement.

# Chapter 11: Distance Healing

You have the symbols in your soul. You have stepped beyond the stage of learning and are now on the path of discovery and limitlessness. What comes next is up to you. The energies involved through the channeling of Reiki by the use of the symbols brings you into direct contact with the Divine. The lessons you learn through the gift of channeling Reiki to others will impact your soul and will bond you to the Universal energies of all and everyone.

Here, in the connection you have gained with this truth and energetic power, you can bring healing energy to the whole of humankind, the earth, and all living beings. Right now, our planet is in a crisis: people are in a state of hate, war, discord, and conflict; global warming is eradicating plant and animal species at a rapid rate; the earth's surface is constantly being plowed and developed by big business. The whole world needs healing.

The level of Reiki that brings the power to healing everywhere is in the power of the symbols. When you allow for Reiki to determine the action and the goal, you can be a power of light to counteract the determination to cause ruin and destruction.

This is the power of distance healing.

Zoom in to the hospital bed of a sick man battling cancer thousands of miles from your hometown. You may have a friend of a friend in need of healing. With permission, you can offer that to him from the comfort of your couch or office.

Harken back to the past of a client who was physically and emotionally abused by a caregiver and has worked for years to find peace and healing, so they can create connections and loving partnerships with others. You can help them by guiding them through their history into that period to channel healing for their abuse.

Look ahead to the wedding of a friend who wants to feel blessed, relaxed, and loved on a special day of bonding and celebration. You can help them beam Reiki to that future moment, to give it the healing, peace, and understanding it needs to be in alignment with the love energy that surrounds us all.

The power of distance healing can cause skepticism and disbelief in many, but the limitless potential of healing like this far outweighs the criticism. The essence of Reiki is in all things: all people, all animals, all plants, all time, all space, all moments. The Second Degree is a much deeper and more powerful understanding of what you can actually do when you are attuned to Reiki. Choose to channel it to help the living.

## Preparations for Reiki Distance Healing

If you are at a point in your Reiki journey where you are ready to explore the possibilities and potential of distance healing, then you will need to practice with great responsibility. Your intuition will be used at an even bigger level; listen to what it tells you about your readiness.

With distance healing, you can send Reiki at will, whenever, wherever, and to whomever. A session can be performed no matter where you are, too. You could be stuck in an airport, traveling to see family during the holidays and have a need to send Reiki to someone else far away. No distraction will prevent you and no location will inhibit you. With practice, you will be able to filter out any and all distractions to perform distance healing.

This naturally comes with second degree attunement, learning of the symbols, and deeper detoxification of yourself as you advance through your Reiki experience. In the beginning, until you feel practiced in distance healing, finding quiet spaces that allow for clarity and focus will help you learn and understand the way distance healing can work.

**Some Guidelines and Instructions for Distance Healing:**

- Give yourself enough time and a quiet space without distractions.
- Predetermine what method you would like to use (more on that ahead).
- Perform a grounding and connection to Reiki energy.
- Let go of the ego to become a pure, clear channel for the Reiki to flow through before you attempt any connection with the person to whom you are sending Reiki.
- Once you feel connected to the Reiki energy, you can begin to transmit it like a radio signal.
- When beginning to practice, try using all of the methods several times each. You may find that you prefer one over others. However, knowledge of each method is valuable and each may be useful in different circumstances. All the methods work, so try them all.
- Use your intuition to determine how long you feel a session should last. This is no different from a regular Reiki session in which the client is in the room with you. The Reiki will travel through you and go where it is needed, continuing to

provide healing even after the session ends. Listen and/or feel carefully into what duration the session should be.
- Typically, a distance session will last for about 15 to 30 minutes, depending on the situation.
- Always use your creative visualization to envision the person, place, or situation with positive light (ex: see them recovering and leaving the hospital; see people dropping their weapons, embracing, and smiling).
- Release all outcomes to the wisdom of the Universe: carry zero expectations of what you think it should be the result. The wisdom of Reiki will decide.
- Once you have performed the session and intuited the end, clearly disconnect yourself from the receiver and ground yourself. Grounding is especially important after distance healing, so you don't get energetically stuck in another place.

## Methods for Sending Distance Healing

It is best for the session that you decide in advance what method you would like to use. Some methods require photographs or props to aid in the treatment, so you will need to determine ahead of time what materials may be needed. This will also help you feel relaxed and focused, so you can maintain clear channeling.

A good rule of thumb is: practice makes permanent. The more you practice each of these methods, the less you will need to refer to any guidelines, allowing for a smooth treatment experience. You may make modifications over time and find that your intuition is the best guide. While learning, keep practicing until you feel comfortable and confident with the methods.

At first, distance healing can feel overwhelming, but the repetition and practice will make it a part of your knowing, permanently encoding into the mechanics of your Reiki channeling so that you will be able to consciously and unconsciously enjoy the experience of distance healing.

You will be using your imagination and creative visualization for almost all distance healing experiences, picturing the person, space, situation, event, or landscape in your mind to perform the function of Reiki channeling to another place or moment in time.

**Surrogate Method**

A surrogate is a substitute or replacement. Since the receiver of Reiki will not be in the same room with you, you can find a physical surrogate on which to perform the treatment. This does not mean another human being. For these types of sessions, using a surrogate means to find an object that you can 'pretend' is the receiver. Most people will use the same object every time they perform a distance healing session. Commonly used surrogate objects include, but are not limited to:

- Stuffed animals, especially teddy bears
- Dolls
- Dummies
- Cushions or pillows
- A drawing on paper of the person
- A photograph (traditional distance healing technique)

What you gain by using a surrogate is that you have a physical representation to stand in as the recipient to help guide you through treatment.

*Note: It is very important to be very clear when you connect to Reiki and begin to channel for a distant recipient that the surrogate is present only as a surrogate for the recipient and not the actual receiver. Stating that in clear terms will be sure to eliminate any confusion and the Reiki will understand what direction to flow.*

For all of the possible surrogates listed above, the idea is that you will actually allow your hands to position themselves on the surrogate as though they are the true recipient. Because you are sending the healing to someone far away and the Reiki is connected to them, you will be guided by the Reiki to direct the energy around the surrogate's form as though it were the true recipient.

Provide a Reiki session to the surrogate as you would the receiver if they were in the same room with you. You will be using all of the symbols for this, projecting them onto the bear or doll, as you would the client.

Practice as often as you can so you can understand the true benefit of using a surrogate.

**Important Note for All Distance Healing Methods:**

State with clarity whenever performing Reiki, and especially with distance healing, that the Reiki being performed 'should be for their highest good.' This caveat makes it clearly understood that you are receptive to the energy knowing where to go and what is needed. You must allow the Reiki to do the work on behalf of the receiver. Always ask permission and state the caveat, or "rider" as it is often called in Reiki.

Since we are not in control of the outcomes or have any say in the best interest of the receiver, we must provide this understanding to the energy and to ourselves. No matter where they are or what they are going through, even if it is a close friend or family member, note that the Reiki be channeled and received should it be for their highest good.

**Thigh and Knee Method**

For this method, you will need a chair to sit in and your imagination. You will be using your knees and the top of your thighs to envision the surrogate.

Your right knee and thigh will represent the front of the body of the person. You will picture the image of the receiver on your leg with their head positioned where your knee is and their feet at the uppermost part of your thigh.

Your left knee and thigh will represent the back of your client's body. The top of their head at the knee and the feet at the uppermost part of your left thigh. You will see an image of their full body as though they were lying face down on your left leg, their body the size it would need to be to fit fully on your leg.

With the symbols, you can accomplish a full Reiki treatment in 15 minutes. You can work on the three positions of the body, head, torso, and legs for 5 minutes each, allowing the Reiki to guide you where it needs to go. Draw, visualize, and imagine the Reiki symbols on the surrogate client pictured on your knees and thighs, being sure to follow the usual protocol of intoning the name of the symbol three times each as they are being drawn and visualized.

This becomes easier with practice and is a great method if you are in areas outside of your home or workspace. You can use it in case of an emergency at the drop of the hat.

### Techniques for Visualization

1. Close your eyes and state your invocation. Connect and ground to the Reiki energy. Repeat the name of your client or friend three times to establish a connection to them. Transport your friend from their sick bed and bring them to the palm of your hand as though they were a miniature individual. See them in your hand when you open your eyes and project and visualize the three symbols onto them from your third eye to theirs, intoning the symbol names three times each. Gently cup your hands around the recipient and keep your hands cupped like this for at least 5 to 10 minutes or until you feel the treatment is complete; the Reiki will tell you. Complete the treatment by grounding and disconnecting.

2. Alternate Visualization: Close your eyes and see yourself in the home or space of the receiver. Have them lie down on their bed or couch in your visualization. Make an invocation and project the symbols, intoning each symbol name three

times as you draw them. Perform a full treatment on the person in this vision. See healing light surrounding them, say farewell and leave them in the healing light, allowing the Reiki to continue its energetic work. Finish the treatment in the normal way, thanking Reiki energy, teachers and masters, and the Divine. Ground and disconnect.

## Traditional Distance Healing Technique

Any time you are performing distance healing, your intuition is incredibly important. Because you are not able to receive feedback from the client's physical or emotional responses when you are with them, you must rely upon your imagination, intuition, and Reiki to help guide you in the correct direction.

### *Step 1:*

Always ask permission. If a person reaches out to you requesting a Reiki treatment, that is your permission. If a request is being made on behalf of another you can do a few things:

1. Refuse to provide treatment without the direct consent of the intended receiver.
2. Use Reiki to contact the higher self of the potential client and ask them the question in your mind if they would like Reiki treatment. Wait for a reply. Reiki will guide you.
3. If the request is urgent on behalf of another and you are unable to receive any input from the potential client, then use your intuition. You will know right away what the appropriate course of action will be.
4. You can also create and send the intention even if a person does not wish to receive Reiki, the energy will go wherever it is needed. Listen to what feels right.

### *Step 2:*

1. Confirm that you have permission.
2. Use a photograph of the receiver that you will hold cupped in your hand.

3. Visualize and intone the Reiki symbols while intoning each symbol name three times as you are drawing them on the photograph:

Cho Ku Rei + Sei Heiki + Cho Ku Rei + Hon Sha Ze Sho Nen + Cho Ku Rei

4. Say the person's name aloud three times as you close your hands around the photograph of the receiver.

5. Imagine being with them, wherever they are. See that person's body in full.

6. Draw the above Reiki symbols again, but on the image of the person's body this time, intoning the symbol names as you do so.

7. Perform a full Reiki treatment in your mind. Pay careful attention to noticeable hot/cold spots or areas that require deeper healing. Use your intuition and Reiki to guide you.

8. End the session as you normally would: comb the aura, ground, disconnect with gratitude.

This traditional format using a photograph and symbols to connect to the client is a guide. You will find that with practice your intuition and intention will always be the best guide for you while you are channeling Reiki.

## Example Uses for Distance Healing

- **Past**: You can use distance healing to repair issues from the past. This is excellent for healing previous experiences, events, and periods of time in a person's life. It will not change history, but it can heal the results from what occurred. People hold onto the past which leads to carrying around a lot of unwanted emotional baggage and blockages. Be clear and specific about where you are going in the past (dates, times, people, situation). It can be a single moment or a whole life period. This is also possible for healing karma from past lives.

- **Present**: You can use the concept of distant healing to help someone's present situation or your own by healing the moment or the immediate future. It is like hitting the refresh button and it encompasses what you already know about healing in the now.

- **Future**: Use distance healing to look to the future, isolating important dates and events, ceremonies, interviews, travel plans, doctor's appointments, exams, and tests, etc. Be specific regarding when. You may go for hours, days, weeks, months, and years ahead. It can serve to help promote the health, wellbeing, and vitality of what is coming up and provide acknowledgement that you are heading in the right direction.
- **Places, World Events, Situations, Disasters**: There is truly no limit to what you can do with distance healing. Use Reiki for healing nature, large conflicts, accidents, war zones, terrorist attacks, political drama, deforestation, animal extinction, habitat revival, crops, ocean pollution—the list continues. Since you cannot get permission from everyone involved in large scale distance healing, it is important to use your intuition and call upon Reiki to guide you and go where it is needed.
- **Multiple People at Once**: You can simply send Reiki to multiple people at once using a couple of easy methods. It's like sending a group email of Reiki energy:

    1. *Reiki Box:* On separate pieces of paper, write down each person's name, situation or event, and details. Include photos as well. Intone and project or physically draw the Reiki symbols on every page, charging each person and situation with Reiki. Close the box and perform Reiki on the box and its contents. Set a time every day to send Reiki in this way.

    2. *Reiki Board:* Similar to the concept of the box, utilize the same method of writing the names of people and situations on separate pages, including photos. Draw and intone the symbols for each person. Pin it to a large board in a secure, private area and

perform Reiki on the board. It is like a vision board for healing others.

*With these methods, it may be beneficial to reach out to any of the individuals that you are sending Reiki to with any feedback you may have energetically received about their situation. Whatever you channel from connection to that energy will help them on their healing path.*

These are only a few examples of the possibilities of distance healing. You are only limited with a lack of imagination and what you discover as you practice this Reiki method. All of its applications will enhance your understanding of Reiki and the Universal Life Force in all things.

# Chapter 12: Conclusion of the Second Degree

Beyond Reiki One, when you are attuned to the Second Degree and receive the symbols, you increase your energetic connection to Reiki. Your abilities are four times stronger than what they are with the level one attunement and practices. This is a huge leap forward and provides you with unlimited abilities to help heal yourself, others, and the world.

The biggest components of the Second Degree are learning the symbols and distance healing. Once you have the symbols incorporated into your Reiki channeling, you should always use them. They enhance every part of the healing process and afford you a stronger connection for channeling this energy to help others.

Distance healing has no end of potential applications. As you start to explore the benefits and possibilities, you will find the beautiful connection we share, bringing each moment to universal and unconditional love. No distance is too great, and time is of no relevance. That is the power of Reiki.

Another major consideration of the Second Degree is permission. Always ask for permission that Reiki be for the person's highest good. Reiki is a living intelligence and knows what to do. Trust the energy and trust your intuition.

The Second Degree is a major transformation on the journey of Reiki. It brings forward a deeper purging a cleansing of your energy and soul so that you may connect as a clear channel to aid others in their healing. The Second Degree brings you into full contact and connection with the Divine source of Universal Life Force and should be treated and greeted with respect and reverence.

When you are attuned in the Second Degree, you will spend at least 1 to 3 years exploring this level of Reiki. For some, becoming a Master comes a lot faster. However, once you are attuned to the Second Degree and the symbols, you must spend quality time practicing, advancing, and exploring. Reiki can take time if you are willing to give. You may be satisfied in your journey once you have reached the Second Degree and feel content to practice healing others from this place.

If your passion is to teach this skill and technique, helping others attune to it, then you will choose to advance to the Third Degree, the level of Reiki Master.

Only you will know what the path holds for you. Trust your intuition and let Reiki be your guide.

# Part 4: The Third Degree

# Chapter 13: Purpose of the Third Degree

Not everyone becomes a Master. Attuning to Reiki in the First and Second Degree does not automatically mean you will advance to the Third Degree: it is a calling. Becoming a Master requires a deep interest in helping others attune to the power of Reiki. It does not mean that you are better, wiser, or more enlightened than everyone who is not a Master; it simply means that you choose to become a teacher so that you can pass the gift of Reiki to others.

Anyone who is attuned to Reiki is attuned by a Master: someone who choses the path of making Reiki their way of life. Many people will feel satisfied with their attunements to the First and Second Degree, content to practice at these levels with the tools afforded by connection to Universal Life Force.

Anyone can become a Master, and only you can determine if it is the right path for you. Having already been attuned for some months or years to the First and Second Degree, you may intuitively know that you need to become a Master, if only just for the reason of helping people attune to it themselves. We all have this energy and this power; we should all use it to heal ourselves, each other, and the Earth. You can help attract people to Reiki so that we can live together in harmony. The more people attune, the better we can all become.

The main prerequisite to becoming a Master is that you must have the intention and desire to help others. Although walking the path of Master is a deeper, more personal, and spiritual journey than any level before, your purpose in the Third Degree is to learn how to attune others to Reiki.

In this level, you will learn the Master symbol which allows you to attune anyone to Reiki, even if they are on the other side of the world. Many of the techniques you learned in the Second Degree will be repeated here, so you will be able to refer back to your knowledge from those chapters to understand the steps involved in the attunements.

In addition to being attuned to a new power symbol when you become a Master, you learn how to use that energetic power to help heal others. You will be able to perform 'psychic surgery' on a client whether they are in the same room with you or on another continent.

Becoming a Master requires a desire and intention to learn more, dig deeper, and truly trust the power of Reiki to heal. As a Master, you are still only a channel for this life force, but you won't need more than your true knowing and trust in Reiki to align with this energy and perform these healing techniques.

# Chapter 14: Understanding the Power of Symbols

You already learned in Part 3 about the symbols of the Second Degree. The power of these symbols demonstrates the potency and meaning behind using symbols to impart energy into our lives. Understanding different kinds of symbols, not just the three available to you in the second level, can help you in your healing approach. Symbols tend to be Universal and also deeply personal. They all have power and meaning, and they can all have an impact, whether subtle or powerful.

There are three groups of symbols:

1. **First Group**: These are called Tattawas. They are simple images that have the power to create an effect shown by the type of symbol used. Example of this are:
   - Yellow Square - represents Earth
   - Blue Circle - represents Air
   - Silver Crescent - represents Water
   - Red Triangle - represents Fire
   - Indigo Oval - represents Spirit

These symbols are very simple and understood across cultures. They are most notably seen in Mandalas which have been used for centuries as pictorial tools to establish focus and centering. The visual shapes, or Tattawas, are said to directly stimulate subconscious energy patterns in the brain. There are thousands of symbols like this throughout history and culture, with a lot of crossover in their meaning and design.

*2.* **Second Group**: They relate to symbolic objects. They are items that can be energetically charged or empowered with intention or ritual. In some cases, certain beliefs suggest that it is enough for an object to be in close proximity to holy places or people in order for the object to absorb and retain this sacred power. Some examples of symbolic objects are:
- Rosary
- Prayer Beads
- Crosses
- Pendants and Medallions
- Crystals, Worry Stones
- Prayer Shawls
- Chalice

Many of these symbols are related to religious practices, but the concept of charging an object with energy is universal.

3. **Third Group**: These are symbols that trigger or ignite awakening. They are considered a light switch for whatever the intention behind the symbol is. Many cultures and religions have such symbols. Reiki symbols provide that spark. Another example is the drawing of a Holy Cross in the air with the fingers during religious ceremonies.

These symbols have the power to:
- Create connection
- Harness energy
- Bring spiritual alignment

- Allow for an opening to accept and receive energy

These are just some of the few possibilities behind power symbols.

## Symbols in Reiki

The symbols of Reiki hold power. Each symbol represents specific energetic properties and function for healing, as well as spiritual amplification. They are each a different way to harness and focus the Reiki energy.

As you learned from the previous section, Usui originally taught Reiki without symbols but brought them into the Reiki teaching to help his students better understand the quality and function of the energy they were channeling. Before the symbols were involved in Usui's lessons, students would receive "Reiju," which was the empowerment from Master Usui to deepen their Reiki connection. At least a year later, you might have been invited to learn and perform Second Degree concepts, but that wasn't a guarantee if you attuned to the first level. Reiki Ryoho was the weekly lesson taught by the master to practice and receive healing treatment.

Times have changed, and so have the Masters. These days, anyone can become a Master if they wish. It is based purely on desire, and you do not have to be invited. You must decide intuitively if it is the right path for you to take.

Further down the lineage of the use of symbols in Reiki teaching, Dr. Hayashi and Madame Takata brought greater focus to the use of the symbols. A new system based on teaching the symbols helped the students learn more quickly due to a greater emphasis on the hand placements and the accompanying symbols.

Attunement was then developed to expedite clearing, connection, and the practice of working with Universal Life Force. Masters trained by Madame Takata were sworn to secrecy about the symbols and other practices.

In our modern world, nothing escapes the internet. We can learn anything, anytime, anywhere, including how Reiki works and what every symbol looks like. Since Reiki is in all of us, we should all be able to utilize its energy.

The use of symbols in Reiki simplified and accelerated the learning process. You already have learned the first three. For the Third Degree Master Level, there is only one symbol, and it is the most powerful of all.

# Chapter 15: Reiki Master Symbol

The only symbol you need to know in the Third Degree is the Master symbol. You will continue to use the other symbols throughout your Reiki practice, and they will always be a part of you, but you will only need to know this final symbol to round out your Reiki power symbols.

### Dai Ko Myo

Pronounced "dye-ko-me-o," this symbol is the most powerful in the group and is only used by a Reiki Master. This symbol's main focus is the healing of the soul and it will bring profound change to someone's life.

It contains three *kanjis*, or characters, which states the mantra "great bright light." To understand the symbol, look at each character separately.

*Dai* – means "big, large, great, or grand" (adj.); can also mean "greatly" (adv.)

## How to Draw the First Character:

1. Vertical line drawn top to bottom.
2. Horizontal line, crosses line 2 left to right.
3. From the bottom of line 1, draw a line out and down to the left at an angle.
4. Repeat Step 3, but draw the line to the right.

*Ko* – means "light" (n.); "purely, completely" (adv.)

## How to Draw the Second Character:

1. Beginning inside the center of the shape drawn by lines 3 and 4, draw a vertical line straight down.
2. To left of line 5 draw a shorter vertical line, slightly curved toward line 5.
3. Repeat Step 6 to the right of line 5, with the line curving toward line 5.
4. Draw a horizontal line from left to right across the bottom of lines 5, 6, and 7. Lines 5, 6, and 7 should be flush with line 8.
5. For lines 9 and 10, you will draw them to look like the mathematical symbol *pi*. Line 9 stems down from line 8, just a little left of the center of line 8 and should curve slightly to the left.
6. Line 10 should begin the same way line 9 does, only slightly right of the center of line 8 and curve much more, almost to a *C* shape.

*Myo* – means "bright, clear, evident" (adj.); can also mean "know, understand" (v.)

## How to Draw the Third Character:

The third character starts underneath lines 9 and 10.

1. At the bottom of line 9, draw a little square.
2. Inside of the square, draw a > symbol.

3. At the bottom of line 10, draw a little square, except on this square you will leave off the bottom line. It will be a box with no bottom.

4. Inside the bottomless square, draw a *z*.

All three characters stacked together bring a message of empowerment, connection with spirit, clarity and recognition about life path, intuition, and creative life force.

Dai Ko Myo is used to initiate and activate attunement of others to Reiki. It is empowering; it opens the receiver to spiritual connection, intuition, and possibly psychic ability. It is very powerful in healing at the cellular and genetic level and is used for even deeper healing of serious illness and disease.

Another function of this symbol is that is shows you your life purpose or vocation. People tend to make dramatic life changes when attuned to this symbol. It is used for the manifestation of dreams, goals, and desires. It resonates with the law of attraction.

It is used in similar fashion to the others. When you want to activate this symbol, you will use the methods outlined in Part 4 for drawing the symbol and intoning its name three times. You can project the image onto your hands or palms while intoning and so the same to the recipient. You will also likely project the symbol onto the crown chakra of the recipient as well as any places that need healing in the body. It works just as the other symbols do, yet it is the most powerful of all.

Dai Ko Myo is not a diploma, degree, or certificate of completion. It isn't even just a simple attunement. It comes with realization, understanding, enlightenment, and the message is strong and clear: there is nothing to attain, there is no goal—just oneness.

Because it represents a greater, more potent meaning and is the first step to letting go of reliance on the symbols so that you are more one with Reiki, you can use the Master symbol in place of all other symbols for any purpose needed.

Dai Ko Myo brings the awareness and truth of the Master: you are Reiki.

## Nontraditional Master Symbols

On your Master journey, you may also learn that there are a number of nontraditional Master symbols that can be used. They are varied and may depend on what Master attunes and teaches you. You can choose to ignore them if you are confident in the traditional symbols, or you may find that here are some with which you naturally connect.

Use your intuition to determine what feels right to you.

A common alternative Master symbol is the *Dumo* (do-moe). It is shaped like a lowercase backward whose tail curls in a spiral with an exaggerated lightning bolt in the upper V-shape. This symbol refers to the swirling, uncoiling fire energy of Kundalini (see Part 1). This symbol is thought to ignite the sacred Kundalini energy that lies dormant in all of us. Since Reiki works directly with all of the chakras, and Kundalini awakens and naturally purges and rebalances the chakras, the symbol is a good fit for this type of energy healing work.

This symbol can be used to pull negative energy out of mental, physical, spiritual, and emotional bodies. It also cleanses and releases energy in spaces, situations, crystals, and anything else you can imagine.

Use your intuition to determine the symbol that brings the most clarity, focus, and connection to Reiki.

# Chapter 16: Attuning Students to Use Reiki

Once you have the Master symbol, you are now capable of attuning students to the energy, whether they are level one, two, or three. You can attune one student at a time or a whole group of students in the same room. You can attune students on the other side of the planet. This chapter will focus on the steps and methods for attuning recipients to the healing energy of Reiki.

## Simple Rules for Attuning Others

1. Students must have intention to become attuned. They must be relaxed and open to receiving the intended attunement.
2. Master must have intention to attune others. They must be relaxed and open to give Reiki to recipients.
3. No jewelry or shoes should be worn by either Master or recipient.

4. Utilize good hygiene principles: clean, odor-free, and hands washed.

5. The student will almost always need to be seated in a chair with hands in a prayer position in front of the heart.

6. Make sure the space is comfortable, warm, relaxing, and has soothing music.

## Steps for the Attunement: First Degree

*For simplicity, the symbols will be abbreviated in the steps. Always assume that if it is written that you will draw a symbol, you will also silently intone the symbol name three times. The two always go together. Any time in the steps it says to draw a symbol this includes intoning three times.*

Cho Ku Rei = **CKR**

Sei Heiki = **SH**

Hon Sha Ze Sho Nen = **HSZSN**

Dai Ko Myo = **DKM**

### *Step 1:*

Ask your student to take a deep breath and have them perform their own, silent invocation about their intention. Once complete, ask that they now relax and listen for instructions.

Begin by drawing a large CKR over the heart chakra of the student. This activates Reiki in the aura.

Cup hands over the heart chakra at a standing distance and beam Reiki into the heart, allowing them to open this chakra to receive Reiki. Hold for at least 10 to 15 seconds.

Walk around counter-clockwise to the back of the student, casting a circle for healing attunement.

*Step 2:*

Move back to the front of the student and stand 2 to 3 feet away. Raise your hands into a prayer and silently invoke a prayer of intention for the highest good of the student.

When you sense Reiki around and in you, you are ready to proceed. Open your eyes and move closer to the student, placing your non-dominant hand on their shoulder. Lift your dominant hand in line with your third eye and above the crown chakra of the student.

Draw the symbols DKM + HSZSN + CKR in the air above the student's crown chakra to call upon and activate the symbols in the ceremony.

*Step 3:*

Move to standing behind the student. Draw a small CKR above their crown to open their crown center. Place cupped hands over the crown and beam the three symbols again, filling the head with Reiki light. DKM + HSZSN + CKR.

Move hands onto shoulders and beam DKM + HSZSN + CKR into their shoulders, arms, chest, torso, thighs, legs, and feet.

Visualize Reiki light flowing through and filling all of the organs, tissues, muscles, and bones throughout the whole body.

*Step 4:*

Stand to the right of the student. Draw a small CKR over the student's throat. With your right hand a few inches from their throat and your left hand a few inches from the back of their neck, beam the three symbols DKM + HSZSN + CKR into the throat, filling it with light.

*Step 5:*

Staying to the right of the student, apply the same technique that you did in Step 4, but move your right and left hand up so that your right hand is a few inches from the third eye and the left hand is a few inches from the back of the head.

*Step 6:*

Stand in front of the student. Draw a CKR over the heart. Cup your hands and hold them side by side, thumbs touching and beam the three symbols DKM + HSZSN + CKR into the heart chakra.

*Step 7:*

Remain in front of the student and draw a small CKR over the student's hands, which

are still resting in a prayer position in front of the chest. This opens the hand chakras.

Place your non-dominant hand around the back of the student's hands, cupping around the thumbs. Gently pull the student's hands toward you. Bend to become eye level with the student, keeping your non-dominant hand cupped around the thumbs. Place your dominant fingertips on top of the student fingertips, so each fingertip between you is matched.

Beam light into the hands and draw the three symbols DKM + HSZSN + CKR into the hands.

*Step 8:*

Leave the student's hands in a prayer position and step back slightly from them. Draw a small CKR in front of the solar plexus chakra, sacral chakra, and root chakra. With hands cupped side by side, thumbs touching, beam the three symbols DKM + HSZSN + CKR into the three chakras and fill the area with light.

*Step 9:*

Move the student's hands to rest in their lap. Draw a large CKR over the front of the student's body to ground their energy.

Place your hands a few inches above their crown chakra within their auric field. Hold your palm parallel to each other over the crown and begin to comb the aura. You will not be touching their body, only their aura. Run your hands down both sides of the aura until you get to the feet.

Touch the floor with both hands to ground you both and to break the connection with the student.

*Step 10:*

Quietly say a Reiki prayer of gratitude. Gently acknowledge to the student that they can open their eyes when they feel ready. Let them know that the attunement is concluded, and they are now attuned to the First Degree, open to use Reiki from now forward.

*Step 11:*

There may be a discussion period after attunement to talk with the student about what they experienced. They may have emotional release during this period and could require comfort during release.

## Steps for Attunement: Second Degree

For the Second-Degree Attunement, you will follow the exact same steps you used for the First Degree. The only modification is in Step 7.

*Step 7:*

*\*\*Modification for the Second Degree\*\**

From Position 6, standing in front of the student, draw a small CKR over the student's hands to open their hand chakras. Gently pull the hands open from prayer and lay them palms up on their lap.

Draw CKR + SH + HSZSN into the palm of the right hand. Intone the symbols three times, but also silently intone that they will stay in the student's hand for life.

Repeat for the left hand.

Help bring the students hands back up to prayer position in front of the heart.

Continue with the rest of the steps from Reiki One attunement.

## Steps for Attunement: Third Degree

For the Third-Degree Attunement, you will follow the exact same steps you used for the First Degree. The only modification is in Step 7.

*Step 7:*

*\*\*Modification for the Third Degree\*\**

From Position 6, standing in front of the student, draw a small CKR over the student's hands to open their hand chakras. Gently pull the hands open from prayer and lay them palms up on the person's lap.

Draw DKM into the palm of the right hand. Intone the symbols three times, but also silently intone that they will stay in the student's hand for life.

Repeat for the left hand.

## Steps for Combination Attunement: First, Second, and Third Degrees

You can combine all three attunements into one session by drawing all four symbols on each palm.

*Step 7:*

*\*\*Modification for Combination Attunement\*\**

From Position 6, standing in front of the student, draw a small CKR over the student's hands to open their hand chakras. Gently pull the hands open from prayer and lay them palms up on their lap.

Draw CKR + SH + HSZSN + DKM into the palm of the right hand. Intone the symbols three times, but also silently intone that they will stay in the student's hand for life.

Repeat for the left hand.

## Crown to Crown Attunement

This is the easiest way to attune someone to Reiki. You will activate all of the symbols above the student's head with the intention set to whatever level they are coming. If they have never been attuned, the intention is First-Degree attunement. Likewise, if they are ready for the Second Degree. You will allow Reiki to take over and channel the attunement on behalf of the student.

As you connect to Reiki through your own body and you become the channel for the energy, your focus and intention will cross from your crown chakra over to the student's crown. The energy will flow this way, from crown to crown, until blockages have been cleared and channels have been able to open, connecting Reiki to the student and permanently bonding them to the use of Reiki. Use your intuition to feel when the attunement is complete.

*Note: Be sure that you make the note in your invocation for the crown to crown attunement that the energy be in harmony with the purpose and highest good of the student.

Every experience is different and unique, and there will be no right or wrong way to experience this. Attunements usually take anywhere from 15 to 30 minutes (some longer).

## Absent or Distant Attunements

Through experience, it has been proven that giving a student an attunement across distance is just as possible and effective as if the student was directly in front of you.

This is an ideal option for people who are unable to travel or have urgent need of attunement.

You will need to have some prior contact with the student via phone, email, or Skype to establish the details of the experience. You will need to explain to them that they are required to study and explore

Reiki on their own. Reiterate the importance of practice, experience, and intuition working on the self and others.

Your phone or email conversation is an opportunity to make sure the student is ready. Provide them regarding how to prepare for the experience and assure that their intention is to be attuned to help the self and others. Let them know about possible side effects that can occur, even with distance attunements:

- Sensations of heat or cold
- Waves of overwhelming love
- May see colors, lights, or symbols
- May hear voices or sounds
- May see people or energy all around
- Intense emotions
- Sense or see past lives
- See or sense spirit guides or passed loved ones

In a distance healing, you will use the Combination Attunement. You will need to decide what Distance Reiki method you intend to use before you perform the attunement (e.g. transmission and/or surrogate, photograph).

Agree with the student about a date and time during your phone consultation. The student needs to have a space and time available that will be free of distraction.

Give them the following basic instructions:

1. Turn off all cell phones and all other devices.
2. Wear loose clothes and remove jewelry and shoes.
3. Avoid junk food, alcohol, coffee, or stimulants for at least 24 hours.
4. Create a comfortable space to lie down or sit. Play soothing music and create ambiance.
5. Mentally prepare prior to the distance attunement through meditation and setting your intention with Reiki. Enter with an open mind and eliminate skepticism.

6. Be ready and relax 5 minutes prior to time you agreed upon, with eyes closed and listening to music.

7. Have a glass of water ready for after the attunement.

Use your intuition to guide you. By Master level, you have likely performed distance healing and the concept applies the same way to distance attunements. The Distance Healing Methods you can use are:

- **Direct Intention:** This connects energetically as though by cords, while light is beamed from you to them through cords. From here, perform the Reiki attunement.

  This usually will occur in the same room, but the distance comes from an inability to get close to the person due to illness or injury, for example. You can also use the Crown to Crown method in this scenario.

- **Surrogate Transmission:** This works exactly like the Surrogate method you learned about in the Second Degree. You can use the same technique with a stuffed animal, cushions, or photograph. You can also use the Knee and Thigh method and picture them on your knees. Again, all the same methods from distance healing apply to distance attunement. The major differences are that you connect with the person to explain the process in detail and make sure they already for attunement and, instead of performing a channeled healing, you give the attunement. (See the Chapter on Distance Healing in Part 3.)

## Psychic Surgery

This tool allows you to go deeply into a serious issue and energetically perform a Reiki surgery to help eliminate stuck, chronic, and various ailments and emotional blockages.

Most of the reason why people are not in their best health is that they attract and create blockages, impeding the flow of life force in their bodies.

Blockages will take on a certain shape, size, color, and lodge in areas of the body and also the chakras and auras. Negative blockages can cause various and serious health issues and other life problems. When the blockages are removed, energy and life force can flow easily.

This is where psychic surgery comes into play. Can be done in addition to a regular Reiki session on the self and others.

***Part 1:***

Give the issue an identity so you can both focus on the clear release of the issue. This can require some conversation during the session. You may also discuss in the intake process. This process occurs in tandem with Part 2.

1. Find the location of the issue. Ask the client to help you know where it is.
2. Determine what it looks like by asking the client what they want to release and heal (it isn't necessary for them to speak it aloud).
3. Ask them to give it a shape (There may be more than one spot. Try to find and work with the main issue. Relieving this first may remove the need to focus on satellite issues).
4. Ask that they give it a color, texture, and weight. Ask if it would make a sound or say anything.
5. Get more specific. Detail brings greater awareness to the problem.
6. Ask them if they are ready and willing to completely let go of the issue.
7. Let them know that you will send it a higher power.
8. Ask them to 'see' the shape they described and focus on letting it go. There is no right or wrong way to do this.

*Part 2:*

1. Try to have the client lying on a table, but you can also do this with them seated.
2. Move behind them and draw DKM on the palm of both your hands.
3. Draw a large DKM down the front of the client's body.
4. Draw a CKR on each of their seven chakras.
5. Visualize your fingers becoming longer, lengthening with energy. Grab a hold of your fingers and thumb of your dominant hand and picture your fingers stretching like taffy as you pull. Your fingers should be about 12 to 18 inches long in your visual image. Breathe and perform finger stretching for each finger. Over time with practice, this will be a very simple and easy technique.
6. Perform the psychic surgery with the full focus and intention. You will use your full being for this: physical, mental, emotional, and spiritual.
7. Say a Reiki prayer.
8. Ask the client to focus on the location of the issue described, adding that they be willing to let it go to be healed. Draw DKM.
9. Use your elongated fingers and the full strength of your being to reach inside the body and grab the negative energy, pull it out and release it to the ground so it can dissipate with Earth energy.
10. Allow your intuition to guide you. Be sure to breathe every time you pull out and release negative energy.
11. Repeat as many times as necessary.
12. Discuss the experience with your client. Ask about the shape, size, texture, etc. Did it change? Did it move? Is it gone?

13. To end the session, step back and make a karate chop movement to cut the cord from the client.
14. Complete a Reiki Gratitude prayer to fully release and ground.

# Chapter 17: Conclusion of the Third Degree

You will never stop learning from Reiki once you are attuned to the Third Degree. Being a Master means you are ready to devote your life to healing. What you offer from the position of Master is an opportunity to share the healing power of Reiki with the whole planet. We are all connected energetically, and this concept is finally understood by the third level of Reiki. The more practice and experience, the more you will witness and feel the miracle of what it can do.

The end of this chapter is not the end of learning and mastering your Reiki skills. There are infinite possibilities for what you can do with this universal energy. Let the end of this chapter be an inspiration to launch into Reiki with new ideas, new inspiration, new energy, and focus. The presence of Reiki in your life will bring you into contact with the truth of the life that exists in us all. Becoming a Master doesn't make you superior to anyone else. It acts as an opening to humbly honor the power of the Universal Life Force that lives in all things and to hand the knowledge to anyone ready for the next step in spiritual enlightenment, whole healing, and sharing the gift with everyone.

We are all one, and we all create this existence together. Be the force of light and love that gently channels the power of healing energy into the hands of others.

*Namaste!*

# Conclusion

Techniques to heal are yours to give. Begin with wholeness on your own journey. Continue practicing healing treatments on yourself to become more attuned and intuitive to the healing connection you now have with Reiki.

If you are a more seasoned practitioner, continue your work holding others through their own healing journey and power. Practice giving Reiki to everything in your life. Offer it to others who are ready to receive healing.

Use it on your cat or dog every day, and watch your plants and flowers benefit from your Reiki channeling. Enrich your food, drink, and living spaces with the healing power of Reiki.

If you desire to become a master and teacher, find a Reiki Master in your community to begin the process of making Reiki a way of life, sharing it with those who are ready to unlock their own true healing power.

As our world continues to change and evolve, so do we. Everything we do has an impact on the health, wellbeing, and harmony of the whole planet. When you bring Reiki energy into your life, you bring it into the lives of others for the benefit of all living things.

Become the healer of your own life and share your understanding of Reiki with those who are ready to awaken to their inner healing power and life force. Take your healing to the next level by getting in contact with all the other Reiki practitioners in your community. Get involved with developing this practice in the world of health and wellness.

Anyone can greet the day with this power and awareness. Reiki is in you and everyone around you. Together, we can heal each other and bring peace and harmony to living things and the planet.

Blessings on your journey!

If you found this book helpful or useful on your journey toward understanding and developing your Reiki skills, please feel free to write a review on Amazon. Thank you for your support.

# Check out more books by Kimberly Moon

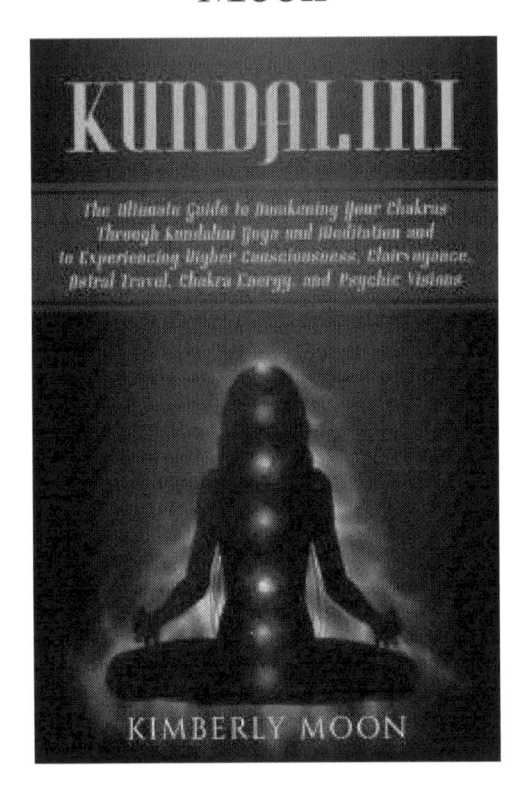

# And another one…

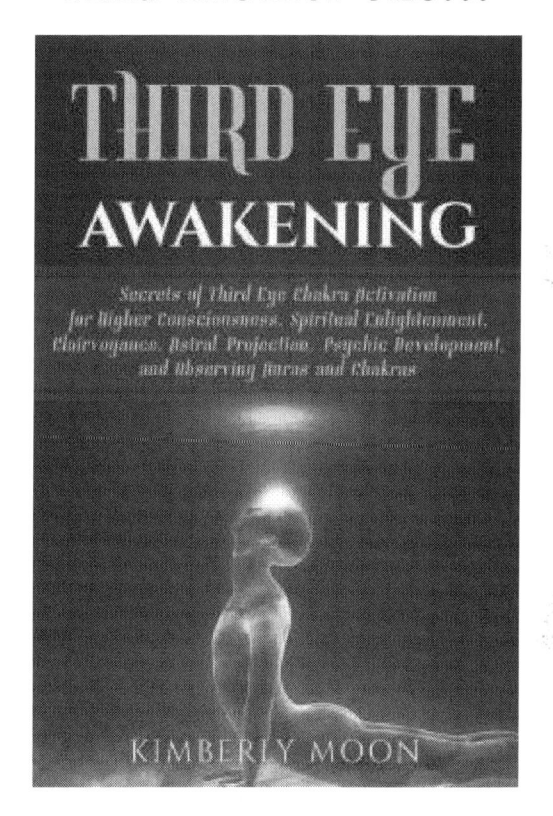

**THIRD EYE AWAKENING**

*Secrets of Third Eye Chakra Activation for Higher Consciousness, Spiritual Enlightenment, Clairvoyance, Astral Projection, Psychic Development, and Observing Auras and Chakras*

KIMBERLY MOON

Printed in Great Britain
by Amazon